Created by Xspurts.com

All rights reserved.

Copyright © 2005 onwards .

By reading this book, you agree to the below Terms and Conditions.

Xspurts.com retains all rights to these products.

No part of this book may be reproduced in any form, by photostat, microfilm, xerography, or any other means, or incorporated into any information retrieval system, electronic or mechanical, without the written permission of Xspurts.com; exceptions are made for brief excerpts used in published reviews.

This publication is designed to provide accurate and authoritative information with regard to the subject matter covered but is for entertainment purposes only. It is sold with the understanding that the publisher is not engaged in rendering legal, accounting, health, relationship or other professional / personal advice. If legal advice or other expert assistance is required, the services of a competent professional should be sought.

♥ A New Zealand Designed Product

Get A Free Book At: https://free.xspurts.com

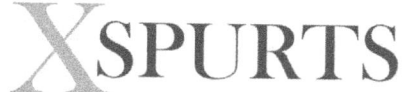

Table of Contents:

Table of Contents:
Understanding Crystal Healing
History of Crystal Healing
Overview of Crystal Therapy
Science vs. Spirituality Behind Crystal Healing
Crystal Selection
Understanding Different Types of Crystals
How to Choose the Right Crystal
Caring for and Cleaning Your Crystals
The Body's Energy and Chakras
Introduction to the Body's Energy Systems
Layout Techniques
Advanced Layout Techniques
Tailoring Layouts to Individual Needs
Meditation and Crystals
Introduction to Crystal Meditation
Techniques for Meditating with Crystals
Benefits of Crystal Meditation
Crystal Healing for Emotional Balance
Crystals for Peace and Tranquility
Crystals for Confidence and Self-Esteem
Crystals for Love and Relationships
Crystal Healing for Physical Well-Being
Crystals for General Health and Wellness
Crystals for Specific Physical Ailments
Using Crystals for Detoxification
Crystal Healing for Mental Clarity
Crystals for Concentration and Memory

- Crystals for Creativity and Inspiration
- Crystals for Stress and Anxiety
- How to Program Your Crystals with Intention
- Techniques for Charging Your Crystals
- Clearing and Resetting Your Crystals
- Crystals in Your Environment
- Crystal Healing Techniques for Pets
- Safety and Precautions when Using Crystals with Children and Animals
- Crystals for Personal Growth
- Using Crystals to Aid in Spiritual Growth
- Crystals for Goal-Setting and Manifestation
- Crystal-divination Practices
- Crystal healing tips:
- Have Questions / Comments?
- Get Another Book Free

Understanding Crystal Healing

Crystals have been used for thousands of years for their believed healing properties. Across different cultures, they are thought to possess energy that can help balance the body, mind, and spirit. The practice of crystal healing involves placing specific stones on the body, surrounding oneself with them, or meditating with them to promote physical, emotional, and spiritual well-being. Although crystal healing has gained modern popularity in holistic wellness practices, its roots trace back to ancient civilizations like the Egyptians, Greeks, and Chinese, who valued stones for their medicinal and metaphysical properties.

Each crystal is believed to have its own unique frequency or vibrational energy. The theory behind crystal healing is that these energies can interact with the human body's energy field, or aura, to bring about healing and harmony. Different crystals are associated with different aspects of health and wellness. For example, amethyst is often linked with spiritual growth and emotional balance, while rose quartz is said to open the heart chakra and promote love and self-compassion.

One of the fundamental principles of crystal healing is the idea of resonance. Crystals are thought to resonate at frequencies that align with the body's natural energy fields. When the body is out of balance—whether due to stress, illness, or negative emotions—the crystal's energy can supposedly help restore balance and harmony. This process is often likened to the way tuning forks can be used to tune a musical instrument, restoring the correct frequency.

For physical ailments, crystal healers may recommend specific stones to target certain conditions. For example, clear quartz is often considered a powerful healing stone for general health and detoxification, while black tourmaline is believed to absorb negative energy and provide protection. On the emotional side, citrine is thought to foster joy and creativity, and lapis lazuli is associated with mental clarity and communication.

Crystal healing is not a substitute for conventional medical treatment, but many people use it as a complementary practice. Research on crystal healing is still limited, and while some studies suggest there may be psychological benefits—such as reduced stress or increased feelings of well-being—scientific consensus on the efficacy of crystal healing remains elusive. The placebo effect is often cited as a contributing factor to the positive results that many individuals report after using crystals.

While skepticism remains, the enduring appeal of crystal healing lies in its holistic approach and its focus on the mind-body connection. Whether one believes in the metaphysical properties of crystals or not, many find comfort in the practice of using stones to foster mindfulness, meditation, and self-care. For those drawn to the practice, the beauty of crystals and the ritual of incorporating them into daily life can also provide a sense of calm and connection to nature's natural elements.

In recent years, the popularity of crystal healing has surged, especially in the wellness and spiritual communities. Crystals are now commonly found in yoga studios, wellness shops, and online markets, where individuals can select stones based on their intentions or needs. Whether used for meditation, energy healing, or simply as decorative pieces, crystals continue to captivate and inspire those seeking to explore alternative methods for enhancing well-being.

History of Crystal Healing

The use of crystals for healing purposes dates back thousands of years, with evidence of their significance found in ancient civilizations across the world. The belief in the metaphysical properties of stones has been part of human culture for millennia, with crystals being revered not only for their beauty but also for their supposed ability to influence health and well-being.

In ancient Egypt, crystal healing was deeply intertwined with spiritual practices. Egyptians used stones like lapis lazuli, turquoise, and carnelian in jewelry, amulets, and as burial items. Lapis lazuli, in particular, was prized for its blue color and was thought to offer protection and promote enlightenment. The famous Egyptian goddess, Hathor, was often depicted with a crystal necklace, symbolizing the importance of stones in spiritual and physical health. Crystals were also placed in tombs, believed to assist the deceased on their journey to the afterlife, further underlining their sacred status.

In ancient Greece, philosophers like Plato believed that the earth was filled with spirits, and gemstones were thought to be an embodiment of these energies. Greek physicians like Hippocrates used crystals in their medical practices, thinking that they could help balance the body's humors and energy. The Greeks also believed that certain stones could heal specific ailments—amethyst, for example, was thought to prevent drunkenness and promote clarity of mind.

The use of crystals for healing extended to ancient China, where jade was regarded as a symbol of purity, wisdom, and health. Chinese emperors and nobles would wear jade jewelry, and it was often used in medicine as a tool for longevity and vitality. Chinese medicine believed that jade could help restore balance within the body's chi (life force energy), and jade rollers have been used for facial care in traditional practices.

In India, crystal healing was embraced by the ancient Ayurvedic and Vedic systems. The Sanskrit word 'Ratna" means gem, and these cultures recognized gemstones as powerful agents of healing. Ayurvedic texts describe the use of stones such as emerald, ruby, and diamond in treatments to balance the doshas (the body's energies). Crystals were also used in rituals to enhance spiritual development and purification.

As we move into the Middle Ages, the use of crystals shifted from a primarily spiritual or medicinal role to being seen as magical and mystical. During this period, alchemists and mystics experimented with stones, believing that they could offer divine wisdom or healing powers when used properly. Crystals were often associated with the stars and planets, with each stone being linked to a specific celestial body and its corresponding influences.

The modern revival of crystal healing began in the 19th and 20th centuries. In the 1800s, the "New Age" movement helped reintroduce interest in crystals and their purported healing powers. Spiritualists, metaphysicists, and energy healers like those involved in theosophy and later in the field of holistic health popularized crystal healing once again. This movement sought to combine ancient traditions with new-age ideas of energy and spirituality, promoting the idea that crystals could harmonize the body's energy fields and provide physical, emotional, and spiritual healing.

Today, crystal healing continues to be practiced by individuals seeking alternative wellness methods. The 1970s saw a surge in interest, with many alternative health practitioners and metaphysical practitioners incorporating crystals into their healing rituals, meditation practices, and therapies. Modern-day healers use crystals in various forms, from raw stones to polished jewelry, and in practices such as Reiki, acupuncture, and chakra balancing.

Although the scientific community has yet to provide definitive evidence supporting the efficacy of crystal healing, the popularity of crystals has only increased. People across the world continue to turn to these stones for their symbolic meanings and as tools for meditation, mindfulness, and healing. The history of crystal healing reveals how deeply human beings have intertwined their physical and spiritual health, and how this ancient practice has endured through the centuries as a symbol of the enduring connection between the earth and the human spirit.

Overview of Crystal Therapy

Crystal therapy is a holistic healing practice that uses the energetic properties of crystals and gemstones to restore balance and promote well-being. Rooted in the idea that everything in the universe, including the human body, is composed of energy, crystal therapy seeks to harmonize the body's energy field by working with the frequencies of specific stones. Proponents of this therapy believe that crystals, with their unique vibrational qualities, can influence the body's energy flow, helping to alleviate physical, emotional, and spiritual imbalances.

In crystal therapy, each type of crystal is thought to resonate with different frequencies, which in turn correspond to different areas of the body and mind. For example, amethyst is commonly used for emotional healing, particularly to calm the mind and enhance spiritual awareness, while citrine is believed to promote positivity and creativity. Each crystal is believed to have specific properties that can be used to address particular issues, whether they involve physical health, emotional turmoil, or spiritual growth.

The therapy generally involves placing crystals on or around the body, either on specific chakra points, energy meridians, or areas that require attention. Crystals are often positioned in a grid pattern, forming a layout designed to amplify their energetic effects. In some practices, individuals might hold crystals during meditation or use them to focus their intentions. Many people also wear crystals as jewelry, using them as an ongoing source of healing energy.

A key principle behind crystal therapy is the belief in energy fields, or "auras," surrounding the body. It is thought that when these energy fields become disrupted or blocked—whether through stress, illness, or emotional struggles—crystals can restore balance. By working with the crystals' frequencies, practitioners aim to remove blockages, rebalance energy, and allow the body's natural healing processes to take place.

For physical ailments, certain crystals are believed to support the body's natural healing mechanisms. For instance, clear quartz is considered a universal healer, thought to enhance the body's immune system and support detoxification. Black tourmaline is believed to provide grounding energy, while rose quartz is often used for emotional healing, particularly for issues related to the heart and relationships.

In addition to their physical uses, crystals are widely employed for their emotional and spiritual benefits. Many people turn to crystal therapy for emotional support, using stones like labradorite or moonstone to encourage introspection, self-reflection, and healing from past trauma. Spiritual seekers may use stones such as selenite to promote spiritual growth, enhance intuition, and clear negative energies.

Crystal therapy is commonly used in combination with other holistic practices such as Reiki, aromatherapy, or acupuncture. Some therapists integrate it with guided meditation or mindfulness exercises, allowing individuals to work with the crystals as part of a larger healing process. The therapy may also be part of rituals or ceremonies designed to enhance personal growth or spiritual awakening.

Though crystal therapy has been widely practiced in holistic and alternative medicine circles, it is important to note that scientific evidence supporting its efficacy remains limited. Many studies on the subject are inconclusive, and much of the healing attributed to crystals can be explained through psychological mechanisms like the placebo effect. However, the popularity of crystal therapy continues to rise, with many people reporting positive experiences and benefits from incorporating crystals into their wellness routines.

Ultimately, crystal therapy is a deeply personal practice, with individuals drawn to specific stones based on intuition, personal beliefs, or guidance from trained practitioners. Whether used for emotional healing, spiritual growth, or physical well-being, crystal therapy offers a unique approach to health and wellness, combining ancient traditions with modern holistic practices. For those who resonate with its teachings, the therapeutic use of crystals can be a transformative tool for healing and self-discovery.

Science vs. Spirituality Behind Crystal Healing

The practice of using crystals for healing blends both scientific curiosity and spiritual belief, creating an intriguing intersection between the tangible and the intangible. While the spiritual community embraces the idea that crystals have metaphysical properties that can influence physical, emotional, and spiritual health, the scientific community remains largely skeptical. The ongoing debate between these two perspectives highlights the complex relationship between science, spirituality, and human well-being.

From a **scientific standpoint**, there is no concrete evidence to support the claims that crystals can directly heal the body or affect its energy field. The energy frequencies that proponents of crystal healing attribute to stones are not measurable by modern scientific instruments. Crystals, made up of minerals and atoms arranged in specific patterns, do have physical properties like color, hardness, and electrical charge, but these properties do not demonstrate any ability to interact with the human body in the way claimed by crystal healing practitioners. For example, some stones like quartz can conduct electricity in specific conditions, but there is no scientific basis to suggest this translates into healing effects on the human body's energy or organs.

Despite the lack of scientific validation, there are some elements of **psychological science** that may help explain why crystal healing seems to work for some individuals. The placebo effect, for instance, is a well-documented phenomenon where a person experiences a perceived improvement in their condition due to their belief in the treatment, even if the treatment itself has no direct therapeutic effect. Crystal healing may harness the power of belief, where the individual's faith in the stone's properties brings about a sense of well-being, calm, or emotional release. This is consistent with the mind-body connection that has been demonstrated in various psychological and medical studies.

On the **spiritual side**, crystal healing is deeply rooted in the idea that everything in the universe is composed of energy, and that living beings are interconnected with the earth's natural forces. Spiritual practitioners believe that crystals, with their unique vibrational frequencies, can interact with the energy field or aura surrounding the human body, helping to restore balance and harmony. In this context, crystals are seen as powerful tools for aligning the body's chakras, clearing blockages, and promoting healing on an energetic level. For many, the act of holding a crystal or meditating with it can serve as a conduit for self-reflection, emotional release, or spiritual growth.

The notion that crystals possess unique healing properties is linked to ancient traditions and metaphysical practices. Ancient cultures such as the Egyptians, Greeks, and Chinese all incorporated crystals into their spiritual and medicinal practices, attributing mystical properties to various stones. This belief system is part of a broader worldview that incorporates energy, intention, and spiritual connectivity—ideas that are often outside the scope of mainstream science but are nevertheless powerful in the lives of those who follow them.

In recent years, **quantum physics** has been cited by some as offering a potential bridge between science and the metaphysical claims of crystal healing. Quantum theory, with its exploration of subatomic particles, energy fields, and wave-particle duality, hints at a universe far more complex than what can be perceived by the naked eye. Some proponents of crystal healing suggest that crystals' atomic structure allows them to tap into this unseen energy, and that their vibrational frequencies might influence the energy fields of the body in ways not yet understood by science. While these ideas are intriguing, they remain speculative and unproven in terms of direct scientific evidence.

One area where science and crystal healing overlap is in the **psychological benefits** of working with crystals. The act of selecting, carrying, or meditating with a crystal can encourage mindfulness, self-awareness, and relaxation—mental states that are widely acknowledged to contribute to emotional healing. Crystals are also often used in conjunction with other healing practices like meditation, yoga, and aromatherapy, which have been shown to reduce stress, improve mood, and enhance overall well-being. In this sense, the ritual of working with crystals can provide a sense of comfort and calm, even if the direct healing effects of the stones themselves are not scientifically proven.

While the **science vs. spirituality debate** surrounding crystal healing remains unresolved, many people continue to turn to crystals for their perceived benefits. Whether viewed through a lens of spiritual energy or psychological self-care, the practice of crystal healing provides individuals with a tool for emotional grounding, stress relief, and personal empowerment. The experience of working with crystals is deeply subjective, and for many, the personal sense of healing they derive from the practice is enough to outweigh the absence of scientific validation. In this way, crystal healing becomes a bridge between personal belief, psychological well-being, and a desire for connection to the natural world.

Crystal Selection

Choosing the right crystal for healing is a deeply personal process that blends intuition, knowledge, and intention. Crystals are believed to possess unique energies that can resonate with different aspects of the body, mind, and spirit. Whether you're seeking emotional balance, physical healing, or spiritual growth, selecting a crystal that aligns with your needs is an essential step in the process of crystal healing. While there is no single formula for choosing the "perfect" stone, there are several approaches to guide the selection process.

One common method for choosing crystals is by their **energy properties** or the specific needs you want to address. Each type of crystal is associated with particular healing properties, which are often linked to the chakra system, the body's energy centers. For example, **amethyst** is widely regarded for its calming and spiritual qualities, making it a popular choice for those seeking emotional balance or greater clarity in meditation. **Rose quartz**, often called the "stone of love," is thought to promote self-love, compassion, and emotional healing, especially when dealing with issues related to the heart chakra.

If physical healing is a primary goal, stones like **clear quartz** are often chosen for their versatility and broad-spectrum healing properties. Clear quartz is thought to amplify energy and is sometimes used to enhance the effectiveness of other crystals. Similarly, **citrine** is believed to promote vitality and abundance, making it a great choice for anyone looking to foster personal growth or career success.

Chakra alignment is another powerful way to choose crystals. The seven main chakras are believed to govern different aspects of your health and well-being, and many crystals are said to resonate with specific chakras. For example, **turquoise** is associated with the throat chakra, helping to enhance communication, while **carnelian** is connected with the sacral chakra and is thought to stimulate creativity and emotional expression. By selecting a crystal that corresponds to a specific chakra, you can work to clear blockages, balance energy, and restore harmony within your body's energy system.

Another approach to crystal selection is to **trust your intuition**. Many crystal enthusiasts believe that crystals have their own unique energetic signature and that the right one will "call" to you. When selecting a crystal, take time to feel its energy. Hold the stone in your hand and pay attention to any sensations or emotions that arise. Do you feel calm, energized, or centered? Sometimes, a particular crystal may simply stand out to you because of its color, texture, or shape, indicating that it's the one you need in that moment.

The **appearance of the crystal** can also offer clues about its energy. Colors are often associated with different emotional and energetic qualities. For example, stones that are red, like **jasper** or **garnet**, are often linked to grounding and vitality, while blue stones like **lapis lazuli** and **aquamarine** are connected with communication and tranquility. Similarly, stones with smooth surfaces might feel gentler to some, while raw, unpolished crystals can carry a more intense, unrefined energy.

Size and shape can also influence a crystal's effectiveness. Smaller stones are often used for personal healing, carrying them in pockets or wearing them as jewelry. Larger crystals, such as clusters or geodes, are commonly placed in spaces to promote a more general, ambient healing energy. Some people prefer the symmetry and precision of polished stones, while others feel a stronger connection to raw, natural crystals, which are believed to have a more direct, unaltered energy.

Purpose and intention are also key factors when selecting a crystal. The energy of a crystal can be directed toward specific goals, such as healing, manifesting intentions, or creating a peaceful environment. If you are working with crystals for manifestation, you might choose stones like **green aventurine** for prosperity or **pyrite** for attracting abundance. For protection, stones like **black tourmaline** or **hematite** are often recommended. When focusing on emotional healing, **selenite** is a popular choice for clearing negative energy and fostering mental clarity.

If you are new to crystals, it's often helpful to start with a few key stones that serve a wide range of healing purposes. **Clear quartz, amethyst,** and **rose quartz** are commonly used in many healing practices due to their versatility and broad spectrum of properties. As you become more familiar with crystal energies, you may feel drawn to specific stones that resonate more deeply with your needs and intentions.

Cleansing and charging your crystals is an important step after selecting them. Crystals can absorb energy from their environment, so it's essential to clear them of any unwanted energy before use. Methods like smudging with sage, placing the crystals in sunlight or moonlight, or using sound vibrations are commonly employed to cleanse and recharge crystals, ensuring they are ready to work with your energy.

Selecting a crystal is ultimately about creating a connection, whether through intuition, appearance, or known healing properties. By considering your personal goals, desires, and sensitivities, you can choose a crystal that supports and enhances your journey toward health, balance, and spiritual growth. Whether you rely on traditional methods, follow your instincts, or both, the right crystal will help facilitate a deeper connection to yourself and the world around you.

Understanding Different Types of Crystals

Crystals are diverse in appearance, structure, and energetic properties, each offering unique benefits for those who seek their healing energies. Whether you're looking for emotional support, spiritual growth, or physical healing, understanding the different types of crystals and their attributes can help guide your selection. These stones are typically classified by their chemical composition, color, and the specific energies they are believed to channel.

Clear Quartz is one of the most widely used crystals in healing practices due to its versatility and powerful amplification properties. Often referred to as the "master healer," clear quartz is believed to help harmonize energy, stimulate the immune system, and enhance clarity and focus. Its transparent, pure form allows it to be used for a variety of purposes, from chakra healing to meditation, and it is often paired with other stones to enhance their effects.

Amethyst, with its striking purple hue, is renowned for its calming and protective qualities. It is often used to alleviate stress, anxiety, and insomnia, promoting a peaceful state of mind. Amethyst is also thought to open and activate the crown chakra, enhancing spiritual awareness and intuition. Many practitioners use amethyst during meditation to foster a deeper connection with higher consciousness or to quiet the mind during stressful situations.

Rose Quartz is best known as the stone of love, commonly used to promote self-love, compassion, and emotional healing. Its gentle pink color is thought to resonate with the heart chakra, helping to release past emotional wounds and open the heart to love and empathy. Rose quartz is particularly beneficial for those healing from relationship issues, grief, or self-acceptance challenges, as it encourages forgiveness and unconditional love.

Citrine, with its bright yellow to golden tones, is associated with abundance, prosperity, and personal power. Known as the "merchant's stone," citrine is often used by those seeking to manifest success, wealth, or creative energy. It is believed to boost confidence, stimulate the solar plexus chakra, and promote optimism and joy. Citrine is also used to help clear negative energy, bringing light and positivity into any environment.

Black Tourmaline is widely regarded for its grounding and protective properties. This stone is thought to absorb negative energies, shield against electromagnetic radiation, and promote stability and protection. Often used in spaces where there is high technology or stress, black tourmaline is commonly placed in homes or workplaces to foster a sense of security and calm. It is also considered a strong protective stone against psychic or energetic attacks.

Lapis Lazuli, a deep blue stone speckled with gold, has been revered for centuries as a symbol of wisdom and truth. Historically used by ancient Egyptians for spiritual growth and enlightenment, lapis lazuli is thought to enhance communication, particularly when speaking one's truth. It is also associated with the third eye chakra, stimulating intuition and mental clarity. Lapis lazuli is often used to facilitate deep meditation and spiritual insight.

Tiger's Eye, with its distinctive bands of golden brown, is known for its grounding and protective qualities. This stone is thought to help boost courage, strength, and confidence while promoting a balanced, grounded energy. Tiger's eye is often used to align the solar plexus chakra and promote mental clarity, making it an ideal stone for decision-making or overcoming challenges.

Selenite is a high-vibrational stone known for its ability to clear blockages and purify energy. Often used for cleansing other crystals, selenite is believed to enhance clarity, mental insight, and spiritual growth. Its clear, translucent appearance makes it especially useful for meditation, helping to clear negative energies and promote a deep sense of peace. Selenite is also thought to connect with higher realms, providing spiritual protection and guidance.

Carnelian is a warm, reddish-orange stone associated with vitality, creativity, and motivation. This stone is believed to stimulate the sacral chakra, encouraging creativity, passion, and emotional well-being. Carnelian is often used to increase energy levels, build confidence, and overcome fear. It's an excellent stone for anyone looking to ignite their passion and achieve their goals.

Hematite, with its metallic sheen, is a powerful grounding stone used to promote stability and protection. Known for its ability to absorb and transform negative energy, hematite is often used during meditation to create a sense of calm and focus. It is also thought to help balance the root chakra, strengthening one's connection to the earth and enhancing physical vitality.

Moonstone, with its ethereal glow, is closely tied to the feminine energy and the moon. Often used for emotional healing, moonstone is thought to encourage emotional balance, intuition, and the nurturing aspects of the self. It is particularly useful during times of transition, such as new beginnings or life changes, helping to align one's energy with the natural cycles of the moon and the rhythm of life.

These are just a few examples of the wide variety of crystals used in healing practices Each crystal offers a unique set of qualities, but it's important to remember that choosing the right one often depends on individual needs and intentions. Whether you're seeking emotional healing, physical well-being, or spiritual enlightenment, the right crystal can help guide you on your journey. Working with crystals involves connecting to their energy, whether through wearing them as jewelry, meditating with them, or placing them in your environment, and it's often a process of intuition and exploration.

How to Choose the Right Crystal

Choosing the right crystal for your personal healing or spiritual needs can feel both exciting and overwhelming due to the vast number of crystals available and their varying properties. While many people rely on intuition, there are also some practical tips and guidelines to help you select the most appropriate stone based on your goals, intentions, and energy.

First and foremost, **clarify your intentions**. Take a moment to think about what you want to achieve with crystal healing. Are you looking to relieve stress, promote emotional healing, enhance creativity, or attract abundance? Identifying your purpose is the first step in choosing a crystal that will resonate with your specific needs. For example, if you're feeling emotionally overwhelmed or heartbroken, **rose quartz** might be an ideal choice due to its soothing energy that promotes self-love and emotional balance. If you're seeking protection or grounding, **black tourmaline** could be the right stone to ward off negative energy and provide stability.

One of the most common methods of choosing a crystal is to **trust your intuition**. Crystals are believed to carry unique vibrational frequencies that can interact with your own energy field. As you explore various crystals, notice which ones you are naturally drawn to. You might be attracted to a particular color, shape, or texture, and this instinctive pull can offer valuable clues as to which crystal best suits you at that moment. Sometimes, the energy of a specific crystal will simply feel comforting or energizing when you hold it. Trust that gut feeling—this is often an indication that the crystal aligns with your current needs.

Color can also serve as a helpful guide when selecting a crystal. Colors are often associated with different emotional and energetic qualities, which can provide insight into the type of healing a particular stone can offer. For instance, blue stones like **lapis lazuli** or **aquamarine** are known to support communication and mental clarity, while green stones like **jade** and **emerald** are linked to heart chakra healing and emotional growth. Yellow and orange stones, such as **citrine** and **carnelian**, often represent joy, creativity, and personal power, making them ideal for boosting energy and manifestation.

Size and **shape** of the crystal also matter. While larger crystals like geodes or clusters can be used to clear energy in a space or for group healing, smaller stones are often more suitable for personal use. You may want a crystal that fits comfortably in your hand, especially if you plan to carry it with you or meditate with it. The shape of the crystal can also influence its energy. For example, polished stones tend to have a more refined, soothing energy, while raw, unpolished crystals are often considered to have a more direct, powerful impact, making them ideal for deep healing or energy work.

Researching the properties of different crystals is another way to make an informed choice. Each type of crystal is associated with specific healing attributes and is believed to influence different areas of your physical, emotional, or spiritual life. For example, if you're struggling with anxiety or stress, **amethyst** is widely regarded for its calming, soothing qualities, while **selenite** is used for cleansing and spiritual clarity. If you're focused on attracting wealth or abundance, **citrine** and **pyrite** are commonly chosen for their associations with prosperity.

Energy clearing is an important consideration when working with crystals. After acquiring a new stone, it's essential to cleanse it of any negative or stagnant energy it may have absorbed, particularly if it has been handled by others before. Common methods for cleansing crystals include smudging them with sage, placing them under running water or leaving them out in the sunlight or moonlight for a few hours. Some people also use sound vibrations (like singing bowls or bells) to cleanse and reset a crystal's energy.

Additionally, it's helpful to consider the **chakra system** when selecting a crystal. Each crystal is often associated with one or more of the seven chakras—energy centers in the body that govern different aspects of physical, emotional, and spiritual health. If you are feeling disconnected or out of balance in a particular area, you might choose a crystal that aligns with the relevant chakra. For example, **carnelian** is linked to the sacral chakra, which governs creativity and emotions, while **amethyst** corresponds with the crown chakra, supporting spiritual growth and connection to higher consciousness.

Finally, **personal experience** is a valuable tool when choosing crystals. If you're new to crystal healing, start with a few basic stones that resonate with you and incorporate them into your daily routine. You might find that over time, your needs change, and you are drawn to different types of stones as you go through various stages of healing and self-discovery. Trust that your relationship with crystals will evolve, and as your energy shifts, you may find new stones that help you on your journey.

Choosing the right crystal is ultimately a blend of knowledge, intuition, and personal resonance. By understanding your goals, listening to your inner guidance, and experimenting with different stones, you can find the crystals that work best for you. Whether you're using them for physical healing, emotional support, or spiritual growth, crystals can serve as powerful tools to help you align with your intentions and enhance your well-being.

Caring for and Cleaning Your Crystals

Proper care and cleaning of your crystals are essential to maintaining their energy and ensuring they continue to serve their healing purposes. Crystals absorb and channel energy, so it's important to cleanse them regularly to remove any negative or stagnant vibrations they may have picked up. Additionally, taking care of your crystals ensures they stay in optimal condition, allowing their natural beauty and energy to shine.

Cleansing your crystals is crucial after you've acquired them, especially if they've been handled by others or exposed to environments where they may have absorbed unwanted energies. There are several methods to cleanse crystals, each suited to different needs and preferences.

One of the most popular methods is **smudging**. Using sacred herbs like sage, palo santo, or sweetgrass, you can gently wave the smoke around your crystal to clear it of negative energy. Simply light the herb bundle, allow it to smolder, and pass the crystal through the smoke for about 30 seconds to a minute, ensuring the energy of the stone is cleansed. Smudging is particularly effective for clearing emotional and energetic blockages.

Running water is another simple and effective way to cleanse your crystals. Hold your stone under cool, running water for a few minutes while focusing on clearing away any negative or stagnant energy. However, be mindful of the crystal's composition—some stones, like selenite and pyrite, should not be exposed to water as they can dissolve or tarnish. If you're unsure, check the properties of the crystal before using water.

Sunlight and moonlight can be used to recharge and cleanse many crystals, especially those like clear quartz, amethyst, and citrine, which thrive in natural light. Simply place the crystals on a windowsill or outside where they can bask in the sunlight or the moonlight for a few hours. While sunlight is energizing and can restore a crystal's vitality, **moonlight**, particularly during the full moon, is gentler and is often considered more appropriate for spiritual and emotional healing stones. Be cautious, however, with crystals like amethyst, as prolonged exposure to direct sunlight may cause fading over time.

Sound cleansing is an excellent method to refresh your crystals and clear stagnant energy. The vibrations of sound waves can be very effective at resetting the energy of crystals. You can use a singing bowl, tuning fork, bell, or even your voice by chanting or singing. Simply play the sound near the crystal, allowing the vibrations to wash over it and shift its energetic field.

Earth burial is another method of cleansing crystals that allows them to naturally release and absorb new energies. For this method, bury the crystal in the earth for 24 hours or up to a few days, depending on the stone. Earth energies are grounding, and this technique is particularly useful for stones like **black tourmaline** or **hematite**, which absorb negative energy and need a reset.

Using other crystals to cleanse your stones is an alternative method. Some crystals, like **selenite**, are believed to have self-cleansing properties. You can place your stones on a piece of selenite overnight to clear them. Similarly, placing stones in a crystal grid with other healing stones can help cleanse and balance the energy of the crystals in the grid.

After cleansing, **charging** your crystals can be just as important. Crystals can hold onto energy from their surroundings, and charging them helps replenish their natural vibrational frequency. You can charge your crystals by placing them in sunlight, moonlight, or even by using a **selenite charging plate**. Some people also use **intention-setting** as a way to charge their crystals—holding the crystal in your hands and visualizing the energy you want it to carry can help reinforce its purpose.

Physical care of your crystals is equally important for maintaining their appearance and energy. Avoid exposing delicate stones to harsh chemicals, extreme temperatures, or physical damage. For example, softer crystals like **sodalite** or **lapis lazuli** can be scratched or chipped easily, so it's a good idea to store them in a safe place where they won't come into contact with harder objects.

For **regular cleaning**, simply wipe your crystals with a soft cloth to remove dust or fingerprints. You can also use a damp cloth for more stubborn marks, but remember not to soak your crystals unless they are known to be water-safe. Avoid using chemical cleaners or abrasive materials, as they can damage the stone and affect its energetic properties.

Finally, consider the **frequency** of cleaning and recharging. Crystals absorb energy constantly as they are used, and their vibrational frequencies may need adjusting. It's generally recommended to cleanse and charge your crystals after significant use, such as following a healing session or when you feel they may be carrying negative energy. Regularly checking in with your crystals—whether intuitively or based on their energetic needs—will help keep their healing potential at its fullest.

By properly caring for and cleaning your crystals, you help maintain their ability to assist in emotional, physical, and spiritual healing. Keeping them energetically clear and physically intact ensures that they can continue to support you on your journey to balance and well-being. Whether you choose smudging, water, sound, or natural methods, find the practices that work best for you, and your crystals will continue to offer their powerful energies when you need them most.

The Body's Energy and Chakras

The human body is not just made up of physical matter; it is also thought to be an intricate network of energetic pathways and centers. These subtle energy systems are believed to influence our overall health, emotional balance, and spiritual well-being. At the core of this system are the **chakras**, energy centers located along the spine, each associated with different physical, emotional, and spiritual aspects of our lives. Understanding these energy centers and their connection to crystal healing can help you maintain balance and well-being in both your physical and energetic body.

There are **seven main chakras** in the human body, each one linked to specific organs, emotions, and energies. The chakras are thought to regulate the flow of energy through the body, and when they are blocked or out of balance, it can lead to physical illness, emotional distress, or spiritual disconnection.

1. **Root Chakra (Muladhara)**
   Located at the base of the spine, the root chakra is the foundation of our energy system. It is associated with feelings of safety, security, and grounding. This chakra governs our basic survival needs, such as food, shelter, and stability. When the root chakra is balanced, we feel grounded, stable, and secure. If it is blocked or out of balance, we may experience feelings of fear, anxiety, or instability. Crystals like **hematite, red jasper**, and **black tourmaline** are often used to balance and strengthen the root chakra, providing grounding and protection.
2. **Sacral Chakra (Svadhisthana)**
   Situated just below the navel, the sacral chakra governs our emotions, creativity, and sexual energy. It is associated with our ability to experience pleasure, intimacy, and emotional expression. A balanced sacral chakra fosters creativity, joy, and healthy relationships, while an imbalanced one can result in emotional blockages, a lack of creativity, or difficulty in forming intimate connections. Crystals such as **carnelian, orange calcite**, and **moonstone** are often used to support this chakra, helping to unlock creative energy and enhance emotional healing.
3. **Solar Plexus Chakra (Manipura)**
   Located in the upper abdomen, the solar plexus chakra is the center of personal power, confidence, and will. This chakra governs our ability to assert ourselves, make decisions, and maintain a strong sense of identity. When balanced, we feel empowered, confident, and motivated. An imbalanced solar plexus chakra can lead to feelings of low self-esteem, indecisiveness, and a lack of control. Crystals

like **citrine**, **yellow jasper**, and **amber** are known to support the solar plexus chakra, boosting self-confidence, willpower, and vitality.

4. **Heart Chakra (Anahata)**
   The heart chakra is located in the center of the chest and is the bridge between the lower and upper chakras. It is the center of love, compassion, and emotional healing. This chakra governs our relationships with ourselves and others, fostering feelings of unconditional love, forgiveness, and empathy. When the heart chakra is balanced, we experience deep emotional connections and a sense of inner peace. If blocked, it can lead to feelings of isolation, sadness, or emotional numbness. **Rose quartz**, **green aventurine**, and **jade** are popular crystals used to heal the heart chakra, promoting love, compassion, and emotional balance.

5. **Throat Chakra (Vishuddha)**
   The throat chakra, located in the throat area, governs communication, self-expression, and truth. It is the energy center responsible for speaking our truth, both to ourselves and others. A balanced throat chakra enables clear, honest communication and the ability to express ourselves authentically. When blocked, it can result in difficulties in communication, a fear of speaking out, or the inability to express one's needs. Crystals like **lapis lazuli**, **aquamarine**, and **turquoise** are used to support the throat chakra, helping to promote clear communication and self-expression.

6. **Third Eye Chakra (Ajna)**
   Located in the center of the forehead, just above the eyes, the third eye chakra is associated with intuition, perception, and wisdom. It is the center of our inner vision, allowing us to access higher states of consciousness and spiritual insight. A balanced third eye chakra enhances intuition, clarity of thought, and the ability to make decisions based on inner wisdom. When out of balance, we may experience confusion, lack of direction, or a disconnection from our intuitive guidance. Crystals like **amethyst**, **lapis lazuli**, and **fluorite** are commonly used to activate and balance the third eye chakra, promoting clarity, spiritual awareness, and intuition.

7. **Crown Chakra (Sahasrara)**
   The crown chakra is located at the top of the head and is the center of spiritual connection, enlightenment, and higher consciousness. It governs our connection to the divine and to universal energy, allowing us to experience a sense of oneness with the universe. When balanced, the crown chakra promotes feelings of peace, spiritual awareness, and inner wisdom. If blocked, we may feel disconnected from our spiritual self or experience a lack of purpose. Crystals like **clear quartz**, **selenite**, and **amethyst** are used to activate and balance the crown chakra, supporting spiritual growth, enlightenment, and connection to higher consciousness.

Each of these energy centers plays a crucial role in our overall well-being, and maintaining their balance is essential for our physical, emotional, and spiritual health.

Crystals work with these energy centers by interacting with the body's electromagnetic field, helping to clear blockages, align the chakras, and restore harmony. By placing crystals on specific chakra points or using them in meditation, you can facilitate the flow of energy, enhance healing, and promote balance in your life.

In addition to using crystals, other methods like meditation, yoga, and breathing exercises can also help maintain the flow of energy through the body and keep the chakras balanced. Regularly checking in with your energy system—whether through self-reflection, energy healing practices, or simply noticing areas of discomfort or imbalance—can help you stay in tune with your body's energetic needs.

Introduction to the Body's Energy Systems

The human body is more than just a physical structure; it is a complex network of energy systems that interact with both the physical and subtle realms. These energy systems are thought to play a key role in maintaining our health, emotional balance, and spiritual well-being. Just as the body requires physical nourishment and care, it also needs regular energetic maintenance to stay in harmony. The most well-known of these energy systems are the **auric field**, **meridians**, and **chakras**, all of which contribute to the flow of energy throughout the body.

At the core of these energy systems is the **aura**, an electromagnetic field that surrounds and extends beyond the physical body. The aura is believed to be a reflection of our physical, emotional, and spiritual health. When the energy within the aura is strong and balanced, it supports the body's health and vitality. However, when the aura is weakened or disrupted by stress, illness, or negative emotions, it can result in imbalances that may manifest as physical ailments or emotional distress. Working with crystals, which carry their own unique energetic vibrations, can help clear blockages and restore balance to the aura, allowing for better energy flow.

The **meridian system**, rooted in traditional Chinese medicine, is another important energy pathway in the body. Meridians are channels through which energy, or "qi" (pronounced "chee"), flows. There are twelve primary meridians, each connected to specific organs and systems of the body. The meridians function similarly to the circulatory system, but instead of carrying blood, they transport vital life energy throughout the body. If the flow of energy is disrupted in these channels, it can lead to physical illness, emotional imbalances, or chronic conditions. Acupuncture and acupressure are popular methods used to balance the meridian system, while crystals can also be applied along specific points to enhance energy flow and support healing.

The **chakra system**, originating from ancient India, is another vital part of the body's energetic makeup. Chakras are centers of energy located along the spine, each governing different aspects of our physical, emotional, and spiritual lives. There are seven primary chakras, starting at the base of the spine and extending to the top of the head. Each chakra is linked to specific organs, glands, emotions, and spiritual qualities. When a chakra is blocked or unbalanced, it can affect the corresponding area of the body or mind, leading to health problems or emotional challenges. Crystals are commonly used to help balance and activate these energy centers by matching their vibrational frequency to that of the chakra in need of healing.

Together, the aura, meridians, and chakras form an intricate and interconnected energy system that influences every aspect of our health. By understanding and working with these systems, we can enhance the body's natural ability to heal itself, maintain a sense of balance, and improve overall well-being. Crystals, with their unique properties, have become a popular tool for enhancing the flow of energy within these systems. They help clear blockages, activate energy centers, and provide healing frequencies that support both physical and emotional health. When used properly, crystals can aid in restoring harmony to these vital energy systems, promoting a holistic approach to health and healing.

Chakras are energy centers within the body that play a vital role in maintaining both physical and emotional health The concept of chakras originates from ancient Indian traditions, particularly within the practice of yoga and meditation. The word "chakra" itself means "wheel" or "disk" in Sanskrit, symbolizing the spinning vortex of energy that each chakra represents. There are seven primary chakras, each located along the spine, and each is linked to different physical, emotional, and spiritual aspects of our lives.

Each chakra is thought to govern specific areas of the body, as well as certain emotional and psychological states. When these energy centers are balanced, we experience good health, emotional well-being, and spiritual clarity. However, when chakras are blocked or out of alignment, it can lead to a range of physical symptoms, emotional imbalances, or spiritual disconnection. By understanding how each chakra functions and using tools like crystals, we can restore balance and support healing in these energy centers.

1. **Root Chakra (Muladhara)**
   Located at the base of the spine, the root chakra is associated with grounding, survival, and security. It governs our relationship to the physical world, including basic needs like food, shelter, and safety. A balanced root chakra provides a strong foundation for the body and mind, making us feel stable and secure. If blocked, we may experience feelings of fear, insecurity, or instability. Crystals like **black tourmaline, hematite,** and **red jasper** are often used to clear blockages in the root chakra, helping to restore feelings of groundedness and protection.
2. **Sacral Chakra (Svadhisthana)**
   Located just below the navel, the sacral chakra governs emotions, creativity, and sexuality. It is the center of emotional expression, pleasure, and sensuality. When balanced, we feel open to experiencing joy, creativity, and healthy relationships. An imbalance can manifest as emotional blockages, a lack of creativity, or difficulties in forming intimate connections. To support the sacral chakra, crystals like **carnelian, orange calcite,** and **moonstone** are often used. These stones help enhance emotional balance, creativity, and a sense of vitality.

3. **Solar Plexus Chakra (Manipura)**
   The solar plexus chakra, located in the upper abdomen, is the seat of personal power, confidence, and will. It governs our ability to make decisions, assert ourselves, and maintain a sense of autonomy. A balanced solar plexus chakra fosters self-confidence, motivation, and a strong sense of identity. When out of balance, we may feel weak, powerless, or struggle with low self-esteem. Crystals like **citrine, amber**, and **yellow jasper** are often used to activate the solar plexus, promoting empowerment and boosting self-esteem.
4. **Heart Chakra (Anahata)**
   The heart chakra is located in the center of the chest and governs love, compassion, and emotional healing. It is the bridge between the physical and spiritual chakras, representing our ability to give and receive love, both for ourselves and others. When balanced, we feel a sense of unconditional love, empathy, and inner peace. Imbalances in the heart chakra can lead to feelings of grief, emotional pain, or difficulty in forming meaningful connections. Crystals like **rose quartz, green aventurine**, and **jade** are commonly used to heal the heart chakra, promoting love, forgiveness, and emotional balance.
5. **Throat Chakra (Vishuddha)**
   The throat chakra, located in the throat, governs communication and self-expression. It is the center of truth, creativity, and the ability to speak authentically. A balanced throat chakra allows for clear, honest communication and the freedom to express oneself without fear. If blocked, it can result in difficulties in communication, fear of speaking out, or a feeling of being misunderstood. Crystals like **lapis lazuli, aquamarine**, and **turquoise** are used to clear blockages in the throat chakra, helping to enhance communication and promote self-expression.
6. **Third Eye Chakra (Ajna)**
   Situated in the center of the forehead, the third eye chakra is the center of intuition, insight, and inner wisdom. It governs our ability to see beyond the physical realm and access higher consciousness. When open and balanced, the third eye allows us to trust our intuition, make clear decisions, and see things from a higher perspective. An imbalance in this chakra may lead to confusion, lack of clarity, or an inability to trust one's inner guidance. Crystals like **amethyst, lapis lazuli**, and **fluorite** are commonly used to activate the third eye chakra, enhancing intuition and spiritual insight.
7. **Crown Chakra (Sahasrara)**
   The crown chakra is located at the top of the head and represents our connection to the divine, the universe, and higher consciousness. It governs spiritual awareness, enlightenment, and the experience of oneness with the cosmos. A balanced crown chakra promotes a sense of peace, deep spiritual connection, and inner wisdom. When blocked or out of balance, we may feel disconnected from our spiritual self or experience a lack of purpose. Crystals like **clear quartz, selenite**, and

amethyst are used to activate and cleanse the crown chakra, fostering spiritual growth and enlightenment.

Each of these chakras plays a unique role in maintaining the body's energy system. When one or more chakras become blocked or imbalanced, it can affect not only the physical body but also our emotional and spiritual well-being. Crystals are thought to help restore balance to the chakras by interacting with their energetic frequencies, helping to clear blockages and facilitate the smooth flow of energy.

Incorporating crystals into your chakra healing practice can be as simple as placing them on the chakra points during meditation or carrying them with you throughout the day. With intention and mindfulness, crystals can help restore harmony to the chakras, supporting your physical, emotional, and spiritual health. Whether you're seeking emotional healing, spiritual clarity, or physical vitality, working with the chakra system and crystals can offer profound benefits for your overall well-being.

Crystals have been used for centuries in various cultures for their healing properties, believed to interact with the human body's energetic systems to restore balance and harmony. One of the most profound ways crystals are used is in conjunction with the **chakra system**. Chakras are energy centers within the body that correspond to specific physical, emotional, and spiritual functions. When these energy centers are in balance, we experience vitality, clarity, and emotional well-being. However, when they are blocked or misaligned, it can lead to physical or emotional distress. Crystals are thought to help restore balance to these chakras by resonating with their unique vibrational frequencies, promoting healing, and clearing blockages.

Each chakra vibrates at its own frequency, which corresponds to a specific color, element, and area of the body. Crystals, which have their own unique molecular structure, vibrational patterns, and energetic properties, are believed to interact with these frequencies. By choosing crystals that correspond to specific chakras, you can enhance the flow of energy in those areas, clear blockages, and restore equilibrium.

For example, the **root chakra**, located at the base of the spine, is associated with grounding, survival, and security. When the root chakra is imbalanced, we may feel anxious, insecure, or disconnected from the world. Crystals like **red jasper, black tourmaline,** and **hematite** are often used to support this chakra because of their deep grounding energies. These stones help stabilize and root energy, offering protection and promoting a sense of security. Their vibrational frequency helps align with the root chakra's energy, restoring balance and fostering feelings of safety and stability.

Moving upward, the **sacral chakra**, located in the lower abdomen, governs creativity, passion, and emotional expression. Crystals such as **carnelian, orange calcite,** and **moonstone** are commonly used to activate and balance the sacral chakra. These stones are known for their stimulating and soothing energies, encouraging creativity, emotional release, and a healthy flow of passion and sensuality. They resonate with the sacral chakra's frequency, helping to dissolve emotional blockages and support the free flow of energy in this area.

The **solar plexus chakra**, located in the upper abdomen, is the seat of personal power, confidence, and will. Crystals like **citrine**, **amber**, and **yellow jasper** are excellent for this energy center. These stones are bright and energizing, offering clarity, strength, and vitality. They work to activate the solar plexus by resonating with its energetic frequency, boosting confidence and helping individuals connect with their inner power. When the solar plexus chakra is balanced, it fosters healthy self-esteem, motivation, and decisiveness.

The **heart chakra**, situated in the center of the chest, governs love, compassion, and emotional healing. When this chakra is blocked, we may experience feelings of emotional pain, isolation, or difficulty in relationships. Crystals such as **rose quartz**, **green aventurine**, and **jade** are commonly used to heal and open the heart chakra. These stones are known for their gentle, loving energies that encourage self-love, compassion, and emotional healing. By aligning with the heart chakra's frequency, these crystals help to release grief, promote forgiveness, and open the heart to unconditional love.

The **throat chakra**, located in the throat area, is the center of communication and self-expression. A blocked throat chakra can lead to difficulty in expressing oneself, fear of speaking out, or a feeling of being misunderstood. Crystals like **lapis lazuli**, **aquamarine**, and **turquoise** are frequently used to activate the throat chakra. These stones are associated with clear communication, creativity, and truth. Their energy helps to align with the throat chakra, facilitating clear, honest expression and empowering individuals to speak their truth.

The **third eye chakra**, located in the center of the forehead, governs intuition, perception, and inner wisdom. When the third eye is blocked, we may feel disconnected from our intuition, experience confusion, or lack clarity in our decision-making. Crystals such as **amethyst**, **lapis lazuli**, and **fluorite** are commonly used to enhance the third eye's energy. These stones have a high vibrational frequency that supports mental clarity, spiritual insight, and intuitive abilities. By aligning with the third eye chakra, these crystals help to open the mind to higher consciousness and intuitive wisdom.

Finally, the **crown chakra**, located at the top of the head, is the center of spiritual connection and enlightenment. When the crown chakra is imbalanced, we may feel disconnected from our higher self, experience a lack of purpose, or feel spiritually ungrounded. Crystals like **clear quartz**, **selenite**, and **amethyst** are used to activate and balance the crown chakra. These stones are highly spiritual, helping to connect us with universal energy, divine consciousness, and inner peace. Their high-frequency vibrations resonate with the crown chakra, promoting spiritual growth, inner wisdom, and a sense of oneness with the universe.

When using crystals for chakra healing, the process can be as simple as placing the stones directly on the corresponding chakra points during meditation or lying down. Some people use crystal grids, combining different stones to create a powerful healing environment. The crystals are left in place for a period of time, allowing their energies to interact with the body's energetic system.

In addition to physical placement, crystals can also be carried with you throughout the day or used in crystal-infused water. The key is to remain mindful and intentional when working with crystals, trusting that their energetic vibrations will help guide you toward balance, healing, and well-being.

Crystals and chakras are intrinsically connected, with each crystal offering a unique vibrational frequency that aligns with and supports the energy flow of the chakras. By using crystals in conjunction with the chakra system, you can promote physical, emotional, and spiritual healing, creating a harmonious balance that enhances your overall health and vitality.

Layout Techniques

When working with crystal healing, the way in which you position and arrange your crystals is just as important as the crystals themselves. **Layout techniques** refer to the various methods used to place crystals on or around the body, to enhance their energetic effects and facilitate healing. These techniques are rooted in the idea that crystals interact with the body's energy field, helping to clear blockages, restore balance, and promote well-being. The placement of crystals is designed to align with the body's **chakras**, energy meridians, or other areas of the body where healing is needed. There are several effective layout techniques used in crystal healing, each with its own benefits.

1. Chakra Layout

The **chakra layout** is one of the most popular and widely used techniques in crystal healing. This layout involves placing specific crystals on or near the body's seven chakra points. Each chakra corresponds to a particular area of the body and is associated with its own color, emotional state, and healing properties. By placing crystals that resonate with each chakra's energy, you can clear blockages, activate or calm the energy of each center, and restore harmony.

- **How to perform it**:
    - Start by lying comfortably on your back.
    - Place a crystal on each of the seven main chakra points, starting with the root chakra at the base of the spine and working your way up to the crown chakra at the top of the head.
    - For example, **red jasper** or **black tourmaline** is ideal for the root chakra, while **amethyst** or **clear quartz** works well for the crown chakra.
    - Relax and focus on the energy flow through your body while the crystals are in place. This layout is usually done for 15-30 minutes.

2. Crystal Grid

A **crystal grid** is a more advanced layout technique that involves arranging multiple crystals in a geometric pattern to amplify their energy. Grids are often used for specific intentions, such as protection, abundance, or spiritual healing. The layout of the grid creates a matrix of energy that supports the desired outcome by harnessing the combined power of the stones.

- **How to perform it**:
  - Start by choosing a specific intention or goal (e.g., healing, manifesting abundance).
  - Select several crystals that align with that intention. For example, for healing, you might choose **rose quartz, amethyst,** and **clear quartz**.
  - Place the crystals in a geometric pattern, such as a circle, square, or star. The center stone is typically the focal point, and the surrounding stones are arranged around it.
  - You can place the grid on a flat surface like a table or altar, or even on your body (if working with smaller stones). Allow the grid to stay in place for an extended period, often for hours or even days.

3. Acupressure Layout

Acupressure layout involves placing crystals on specific points of the body that correspond to acupressure points or meridian pathways. This technique is inspired by traditional Chinese medicine and the understanding that energy flows through the body's meridians. By applying crystals to these points, you can help restore the flow of **qi** (life force energy), clear blockages, and support physical and emotional healing.

- **How to perform it**
  - Choose a selection of crystals that correspond to the meridian points or acupressure zones you wish to work on.
  - Common meridian points include areas like the wrists, behind the knees, and the soles of the feet.
  - Place the crystals on or near these points, either directly on the skin or just above the area, depending on your comfort level.
  - Hold the crystals in place for several minutes while you focus on the intention of restoring balance and healing energy flow.

4. The Crystal Healing Circle

The **crystal healing circle** is an arrangement where you sit or lie in the center of a circle made from crystals. This layout is designed to create a powerful energy field around you, providing protection, support, and healing. The circle can be composed of any type of crystals, and it is often used for grounding or meditative practices.

- **How to perform it**:
  - Arrange a circle of crystals on the floor around you. The size of the circle can vary, but it should be large enough to surround you comfortably.
  - The crystals can be placed at equal intervals, and you may want to use larger stones or specific types like **black tourmaline** for protection, or **amethyst** for spiritual connection.

- Once you are inside the circle, relax, close your eyes, and focus on your breathing. Allow the crystals to work with your energy field, promoting a sense of peace and grounding.

5. Crystal Bath

A **crystal bath** is a more immersive method of working with crystals and involves placing them in a bath or using them in combination with water to cleanse and rejuvenate the body. This layout technique can be done with either large or small crystals that can be safely placed in the water. The idea is that the water amplifies the energetic properties of the crystals, allowing them to cleanse, refresh, and heal.

- **How to perform it**:
    - Choose crystals that are safe to use in water, such as **amethyst, rose quartz**, or **clear quartz**.
    - Place the crystals in your bathwater and soak for at least 20 minutes.
    - As you relax, focus on the intention of releasing negativity, balancing your energy, and rejuvenating your spirit.

6. The Pendulum Layout

Using a pendulum in conjunction with crystal layouts is an effective method to test energy flow and identify blockages in the body. Pendulums can be made from crystals themselves, or they can be used in combination with stones to gauge energy alignment.

- **How to perform it**:
    - Hold a crystal pendulum above your body or specific chakra points.
    - Observe the direction and speed of the pendulum's movement. A clockwise motion is often seen as a sign of energy flow, while a counterclockwise motion may indicate a blockage.
    - Once you've identified areas of imbalance, place the appropriate crystals on those spots to restore energy flow.

Conclusion

In crystal healing, the way crystals are arranged and placed is essential to achieving their full healing potential. Whether using a **chakra layout** to align energy centers, creating a **crystal grid** to manifest specific intentions, or forming a **healing circle** for protection and grounding, each layout technique offers a unique way to interact with the crystals' energy. By experimenting with different layouts, you can discover which works best for your personal healing journey and enhance your well-being in a deeper, more intentional way.

Crystal grids and layouts are powerful tools in the practice of crystal healing, designed to amplify the energies of the stones and direct them toward specific healing intentions. These techniques involve strategically placing crystals in geometric patterns, creating a network of energy that interacts with your body's own energetic field. Whether used for personal healing, manifestation, or spiritual growth, crystal grids harness the power of sacred geometry to enhance the effects of the stones.

The concept behind crystal grids is rooted in the belief that the arrangement of stones in certain shapes or patterns can create a unified, focused energy that enhances the vibrational frequency of the crystals. The most common geometric patterns used in crystal grids include the **Flower of Life**, **Sacred Geometry**, **Merkaba**, and **Hexagonal** formations. These shapes are thought to align with the natural laws of the universe and can direct energy in a specific way. The layout of the grid helps activate the intention behind it, whether that's healing, abundance, protection, or clarity.

1. Setting an Intention

The first and most important step in creating a crystal grid is setting a clear intention. The energy of the grid is directly influenced by the intention you place upon it. Whether your goal is to heal emotional wounds, manifest prosperity, or create peace, the energy of the crystals will work in alignment with your purpose. Be specific about your intention and focus on it throughout the process.

To begin, choose your desired outcome and hold that thought clearly in your mind. You may also wish to write down your intention on a piece of paper or use words or symbols to represent your goals. This intention will serve as the foundation for the energy you're about to direct.

2. Choosing Crystals

Once your intention is clear, it's time to select the crystals that will support it. Different stones carry unique energies that correspond to various aspects of life, such as emotional healing, physical health, abundance, or spiritual growth. Here are some examples of crystals and their associated properties:

- **Clear Quartz**: Amplifies energy, clears blockages, and enhances overall healing.
- **Amethyst**: Used for spiritual growth, intuition, and calming the mind.
- **Rose Quartz**: Promotes love, emotional healing, and self-compassion.
- **Citrine**: Attracts abundance, prosperity, and personal power.
- **Black Tourmaline**: Offers protection, grounding, and energetic cleansing.

The key is to select crystals that align with the specific intention of your grid. You may also choose a central crystal or "master stone," which serves as the focal point of the grid, while surrounding stones (often in smaller sizes) amplify its energy.

3. Choosing the Grid Layout

The arrangement of the crystals is crucial for the success of the grid. Sacred geometry plays a central role in how the energy will be directed and expanded. Here are some common layouts:

- **The Flower of Life**: A symbol of divine creation and spiritual enlightenment, this grid is often used for manifesting abundance, personal growth, or higher consciousness. It involves multiple overlapping circles, each representing a different aspect of life, creating a beautiful web of interconnected energy.
- **The Merkaba**: Known as the sacred geometric shape of light, the Merkaba is a star tetrahedron that is used to connect with higher spiritual realms, promote deep meditation, or facilitate transformative energy. It is especially helpful for those seeking to activate the third eye or crown chakras.
- **The Hexagonal Grid**: The hexagon is a powerful shape that represents balance, harmony, and unity. This layout is ideal for grounding, protection, and emotional healing. The symmetry of the hexagon is thought to support the flow of energy in a balanced and harmonious way.
- **The Spiral**: The spiral pattern represents the flow of life, evolution, and expansion. It's often used for personal transformation and healing journeys. This shape allows energy to move outward, supporting growth and the unfolding of new opportunities.
- **The Square or Rectangle**: Known for providing stability and structure, these grids are commonly used for creating balance and order in life. This layout is helpful when seeking to manifest material goals or enhance practical achievements.

4. Placing the Crystals

After selecting your crystals and determining your grid layout, it's time to place the stones in the chosen pattern. Start with the central stone, the anchor of your intention, and build outward, placing the surrounding crystals one by one, working in a clockwise direction to activate the grid. Some people prefer to cleanse their crystals before beginning, either by using smoke, sound, or visualization, to ensure the stones are free of any lingering or negative energy.

- **Central Stone**: This is typically the most significant crystal and is placed in the center of the grid. It serves as the "master" stone that amplifies and directs the energy.
- **Surrounding Stones**: Place the surrounding crystals strategically, paying attention to how their energies might complement each other. Consider the energetic properties of each stone and how they will support your intention.
- **Activation**: Once the grid is complete, it's time to activate it. This is often done by holding a **clear quartz** or another point crystal and directing energy from the

crystal over the grid. You may also choose to visualize a beam of light activating the grid or gently tracing the pattern of the grid with your hand to symbolically "activate" the energy flow. Alternatively, some practitioners prefer to focus their breath, sending intention and energy through their breath to bring the grid to life.

5. Using the Grid

Once the grid is set up and activated, the work isn't necessarily over. The energy of the grid continues to work, so it's important to spend time near it to connect with the vibrations of the stones. This can be done by sitting or lying near the grid, meditating, or simply focusing on your intention and breathing. The grid can be left in place for a period of time—usually a few days or even weeks—while the energy is being absorbed by the crystals and directed toward the intended outcome.

You may also choose to update or refresh the grid by adding new crystals, shifting the layout, or reactivating it with new energy as your goals evolve.

6. Clearing the Grid

After the grid has served its purpose, it's important to clear the energy. This can be done by gently removing each crystal from the grid, thanking them for their support, and cleansing them for future use. You can also reset the grid by re-aligning the stones or creating a new layout when you're ready to set a new intention.

Crystal grids are a beautiful, intentional way to harness the power of crystals and direct their healing energy toward a desired goal. By carefully selecting crystals, aligning them in sacred geometric patterns, and focusing on a clear intention, you can amplify your healing practice and work with the energy of the earth to manifest your desires.

Advanced Layout Techniques

When you've mastered the basics of crystal layouts, there are several advanced techniques that can deepen the effectiveness of your healing practices. These methods often involve more complex arrangements and can be tailored to specific needs, such as heightened spiritual awareness, deep emotional healing, or energetic protection. By applying advanced layout techniques, you can create powerful energetic structures that amplify the crystals' natural properties and facilitate more profound healing experiences.

1. Sacred Geometry Grid Layouts

Sacred geometry is a central element in advanced crystal layout techniques. These geometric patterns are based on universal laws of harmony and balance, and they are believed to resonate with the natural frequencies of the earth and the cosmos. Crystals placed within these patterns are thought to align energies in a way that fosters deep healing, spiritual awakening, and transformation.

Flower of Life Grid: One of the most famous sacred geometry patterns, the Flower of Life represents the interconnectedness of all life. It consists of overlapping circles arranged to create a pattern of symmetrical shapes. This grid is used to amplify universal energy, promote spiritual awakening, and enhance personal growth. The symmetry of the Flower of Life encourages balance in all aspects of life, and its energetic signature is especially beneficial for those seeking alignment with the cosmos.

Merkaba Grid: The Merkaba is a star tetrahedron, a three-dimensional figure formed by two interlocking pyramids. In crystal healing, the Merkaba grid is used to activate and balance the light body. It is often employed for spiritual protection, meditation, and advanced healing practices. This grid is thought to connect the physical body with higher realms of consciousness and assist in soul-level healing.

Golden Ratio Spiral: Based on the Fibonacci sequence, this spiral shape is another form of sacred geometry used in advanced grids. The Golden Ratio spiral, or Phi Spiral, is a symbol of growth, harmony, and transformation. Crystals arranged in this pattern are thought to facilitate expansion in consciousness and encourage natural flow in the healing process.

2. Crystal Circuitry Layout

Crystal circuiting involves creating a flow of energy by arranging crystals in a network that forms an energetic circuit. The goal of this technique is to channel energy more effectively through the body or an environment. It's commonly used to clear energy blockages, energize the meridians, or align the body's energy field.

How to create a crystal circuit:

- Select a combination of stones that correspond to specific chakras or energy points.
- Arrange the stones in a continuous loop, either around the body or in a room, to form a circuit. Typically, you'd place one stone at each chakra or energy point.
- The stones should be aligned to create an unbroken energy flow. If you're creating a circuit around your body, you could place crystals at the feet, hands, and over the heart, with other stones creating a loop that aligns with the energy centers.

This technique can be used to increase vitality, enhance focus, or clear energetic imbalances that hinder the natural flow of energy in the body.

3. Crystal and Light Therapy Layouts

In advanced crystal healing, light therapy can be combined with crystal layouts to increase the healing potential. By using crystals in combination with natural light or colored light, you can target specific energy points in the body, stimulating healing and transformation. The practice of crystal and light therapy is particularly effective when using crystals known to amplify or transmit light, such as **clear quartz, selenite, and amethyst**.

How to use light in crystal layouts:

- Place the crystals in a space where natural light enters (like by a window) or use a light source such as a lamp with colored bulbs.
- Align crystals in a pattern that corresponds to the chakras or energy points you wish to work on.
- Focus on the way the light interacts with the crystals. For instance, sunlight passing through a clear quartz point can amplify its energy and send a stream of light directly to the body, activating healing in the designated area.

Colored light (such as red, blue, or violet) can be used in combination with specific crystals to further balance and support the energy of the chakras.

4. Crystal Layering Layouts

Crystal layering involves stacking or placing crystals on top of each other to amplify their healing properties. By layering different stones that correspond to various healing needs, you create a composite energetic effect that targets multiple levels of healing at once. This technique is particularly effective when you need to address more complex or multifaceted issues, such as deep emotional trauma, spiritual blockage, or chronic physical ailments.

How to layer crystals:

- Choose stones that address different layers of an issue. For example, if you're working on emotional healing, you could layer **rose quartz** (for love and emotional healing) with **black tourmaline** (for protection and grounding).
- Stack smaller stones over larger ones or place them next to each other. You may also want to place a crystal directly on top of the corresponding chakra point.
- The key with layering is to balance the stones with complementary properties. Each crystal should support the healing intention and help create a harmonious energetic flow.

This technique works by creating a stronger vibrational field that addresses the root causes of imbalances and facilitates deeper transformation.

5. Geometric Activations for Advanced Healing

Geometric activation involves using highly specific geometric formations to bring energy into an area of the body or space that requires healing. This practice goes beyond simply placing crystals in a shape; it involves intentional activation of specific energy grids within the body using both crystals and visualization.

Activation Process:

- Choose a sacred geometry pattern (such as the **Merkaba, Flower of Life**, or **Hexagonal grid**).
- Place stones on the body, on the ground, or in the environment according to the geometric pattern, ensuring that the stones are aligned with the energy centers you intend to activate.
- Visualize the energetic lines of the pattern connecting each stone, forming a web of interconnected energy. Focus on sending your intention into the grid, directing healing energy to the areas in need.
- This technique is most powerful when combined with breathwork or meditation, as these practices help to open the energy channels and allow the geometric shape to activate deeper levels of healing.

6. Crystal Amplification Layouts

Crystal amplification is used when you need to enhance a particular energy in a specific area of your life. The idea is to use larger stones or certain highly energetic crystals to boost the power of the smaller, less intense stones placed nearby. This layout works by amplifying the intention and energy of specific stones, helping to direct or increase the energy flow in targeted areas.

How to amplify energy:

- Choose a large crystal that resonates with your specific intention (e.g., **clear quartz, amethyst, or selenite**).
- Surround this central stone with smaller, more focused crystals that carry similar or complementary energies.
- For example, you might use a **large citrine** to amplify the energy of prosperity and place smaller stones such as **green aventurine** or **pyrite** around it to further draw in abundance.

By strategically amplifying certain energies, you can greatly enhance the effectiveness of your healing sessions and ensure that the energy is directed exactly where it's needed most.

7. Healing Through the Elements Layout

Each element—earth, water, fire, and air—corresponds to different energies within the body and nature. By using crystal layouts that align with these elements, you can enhance healing in specific areas of your life or body.

- **Earth**: Grounding, stability, and security (e.g., **hematite, black tourmaline**)
- **Water**: Emotional healing, fluidity, and creativity (e.g., **moonstone, aquamarine**)
- **Fire**: Transformation, passion, and personal power (e.g., **citrine, red jasper**)
- **Air**: Mental clarity, communication, and higher consciousness (e.g., **clear quartz, sodalite**)

Place stones that resonate with each element on their respective areas of the body or room to harmonize with and strengthen the corresponding elemental energies.

Conclusion

Advanced crystal layout techniques open up a vast array of possibilities for deeper healing and energetic alignment. By incorporating sacred geometry, crystal circuiting, light therapy, and geometric activation into your practice, you can enhance the effects of crystal healing and target specific intentions more effectively. These advanced techniques require focus, intention, and awareness, but they offer powerful ways to amplify the healing potential of crystals and create transformative changes in your life.

Tailoring Layouts to Individual Needs

When working with crystals, it's important to tailor your layouts to the specific needs of the individual or situation. Each person has unique energy requirements, and customizing the crystal layout allows for more effective healing. Whether you're addressing emotional imbalances, physical ailments, or spiritual growth, the right arrangement of crystals can target the areas that need attention, enhancing their healing potential.

1. Tailoring for Emotional Healing

For those seeking emotional healing or relief from stress and anxiety, choosing crystals that promote peace, calm, and emotional balance is key. **Rose quartz**, known as the stone of unconditional love, is an excellent choice for fostering compassion and emotional healing. Pairing it with **amethyst** can help soothe stress and promote a peaceful, meditative state. Crystals like **black tourmaline** can be added for protection, especially if negative emotional energy needs to be cleared.

Layout Tips:

- Place **rose quartz** over the heart chakra to encourage self-love and emotional healing.
- **Amethyst** can be placed on the forehead (third eye) to calm the mind and enhance emotional clarity.
- Arrange **black tourmaline** at the corners of the space to protect against negative energies.

This layout can be done as a grid on a meditation mat or while lying down, ensuring the stones are placed directly over the corresponding chakras.

2. Tailoring for Physical Healing

Physical ailments often require specific crystal types that target particular body areas or organ systems. **Hematite**, known for its grounding and blood-purifying properties, is useful for circulatory issues and grounding energy. **Carnelian** is excellent for boosting energy and vitality, while **selenite** can help clear blocked energy in the body.

Layout Tips:

- **Amethyst** can be placed over areas of pain or discomfort to alleviate tension and promote relaxation.
- **Clear quartz** can amplify the healing properties of any other crystal and can be placed over the area where healing is needed.
- Create a crystal circuit or grid around the body, starting with grounding stones like **hematite** at the feet and working your way up with stones that correspond to specific ailments.

Focus on the areas of the body where healing is most needed and ensure the crystal's energy aligns with the root cause of the issue.

3. Tailoring for Mental Clarity and Focus

For mental clarity, concentration, and focus, certain crystals can stimulate the mind and promote clear thought. **Citrine**, with its bright energy, enhances focus and stimulates mental clarity, while **fluorite** can assist in clearing mental fog and aiding decision-making. **Sodalite** is also helpful for communication and self-expression, especially when needing to clarify thoughts or articulate ideas.

Layout Tips:

- Place **sodalite** over the throat chakra to support clear communication and mental articulation.
- Position **fluorite** on the third eye chakra (forehead) to help clear mental blockages and enhance intuition.
- Use **citrine** on the solar plexus to energize the mind and stimulate focus.

A simple grid placed in a circle around the head or on a meditation table can help amplify these effects, allowing the crystals to clear the mind and sharpen focus.

4. Tailoring for Spiritual Growth

For spiritual growth, enlightenment, and higher consciousness, crystals that resonate with the upper chakras—such as the third eye and crown chakras—are essential. **Amethyst** enhances spiritual awareness and intuition, while **clear quartz** serves as a powerful amplifier for any energy. **Labradorite** is excellent for accessing deeper layers of consciousness, and **sodalite** can aid in connecting with the higher self.

Layout Tips:

- Place **amethyst** on the third eye to enhance intuition and psychic awareness.
- **Clear quartz** can be placed at the crown chakra to support spiritual connection and enlightenment.

- Arrange **labradorite** around the body to form a protective spiritual shield while opening up the connection to higher realms.

These layouts work well for meditation, where the person can focus on their spiritual intentions, allowing the crystals to guide their inner journey.

5. Tailoring for Protection

Protection layouts are especially useful when shielding from negative energies or when in need of emotional or energetic defense. **Black tourmaline** is the go-to stone for grounding and protection, while **obsidian** can cut through negativity and shield from unwanted energies. **Shungite** is known for its protective qualities against electromagnetic fields and environmental toxins.

Layout Tips:

- Place **black tourmaline** at the corners of your space to create a protective grid.
- **Obsidian** can be placed on the root chakra or near the feet for grounding protection.
- Create a shield by arranging **shungite** around your workspace or meditation area, ensuring it forms a boundary around you.

Protection layouts should be designed to form a perimeter around the person or space, creating a solid energetic shield from unwanted influences.

6. Tailoring for Manifestation

Manifestation layouts are intended to help bring desires or intentions into reality, often with the help of crystals that promote abundance and the power of attraction. **Citrine and pyrite** are excellent for manifesting wealth and success, while **green aventurine** supports luck and opportunities. **Tiger's eye** enhances personal power and confidence, crucial for manifesting your goals.

Layout Tips:

- Use **citrine** at the solar plexus chakra to amplify personal willpower and attract success.
- Place **green aventurine** over the heart chakra to open the heart to abundance and opportunities.
- **Pyrite** can be placed near the front door or entrance to draw in prosperity and good fortune.

A crystal grid formed in a geometric shape, such as a square or diamond, is ideal for directing focused energy into manifestation goals.

7. Tailoring for Grounding

Grounding layouts help to anchor and stabilize the body's energy, especially for those who feel scattered or disconnected. **Hematite** is one of the best stones for grounding, as it connects the root chakra with the earth's stabilizing energy. **Smoky quartz** is also effective in transmuting negative energy into positive energy, while **red jasper** brings a nurturing and stabilizing influence.

Layout Tips:

- Place **hematite** on the feet or the root chakra to ground energy and provide stability.
- Position **red jasper** over the sacral chakra to stabilize emotional energy and support creativity.
- Arrange **smoky quartz** at the base of the spine to clear negative energy and restore balance.

This layout can be performed while sitting or lying down, focusing on breathing and visualizing yourself connected to the earth.

Conclusion

Tailoring crystal layouts to individual needs involves selecting the right stones for specific goals and arranging them in ways that maximize their energetic properties. Whether you're seeking emotional balance, physical healing, mental clarity, spiritual growth, or protection, custom layouts allow for a deeper, more targeted healing experience. By considering the specific needs of the individual or situation, and combining the power of different crystals in carefully crafted arrangements, you can enhance the effectiveness of crystal healing and help manifest desired outcomes.

Meditation and Crystals

Meditation is a powerful practice that allows the mind to become still and focused, promoting clarity, relaxation, and spiritual growth. When combined with crystals, meditation becomes an even more profound and transformative experience. Crystals, with their unique energy vibrations, can enhance meditation by helping to clear energetic blockages, deepen concentration, and connect with higher states of consciousness. By choosing the right crystals and incorporating them into your meditation practice, you can amplify the benefits and achieve deeper levels of relaxation and insight.

1. Choosing the Right Crystal for Meditation

Each crystal has its own energy and healing properties, and selecting the right one for meditation can enhance the specific intention or goal of your session. For instance, if you're seeking peace and emotional healing, **rose quartz** may be the ideal stone. If you wish to enhance intuition and spiritual connection, **amethyst** or **lapis lazuli** may be more suitable. The key is to select a crystal that resonates with your needs and goals.

- **Amethyst**: Known for its calming and spiritual properties, amethyst is ideal for meditation aimed at stress relief, spiritual growth, and deepening intuition.
- **Clear Quartz**: This stone is often referred to as the "master healer" because it amplifies energy. It's ideal for enhancing mental clarity and meditation focused on healing and balance.
- **Citrine**: A stone of abundance and manifestation, citrine is great for meditation practices aimed at manifesting goals and enhancing personal power.
- **Selenite**: Known for its purifying and cleansing properties, selenite can help clear negative energy and create a peaceful environment for deep meditation.
- **Labradorite**: Perfect for connecting with higher realms and enhancing spiritual exploration, labradorite is often used in meditations focused on personal transformation and self-discovery.

2. How to Use Crystals in Meditation

There are several ways to incorporate crystals into your meditation practice. The method you choose will depend on your intention and how you feel the crystals work best for you. Here are a few ways to use crystals during meditation:

Holding Crystals

One of the simplest ways to use crystals in meditation is to hold them in your hands. Placing a crystal in each hand or one in your dominant hand allows the energy to flow directly into your energy field. As you meditate, focus on the sensations the crystal is creating, whether it is warmth, tingling, or a sense of calm. For example, holding **rose quartz** can promote feelings of love and emotional healing, while **amethyst** can soothe the mind and promote spiritual awareness.

Placing Crystals on the Body

Another popular technique is to place crystals on the body, particularly at energy centers such as the chakras. For example, placing **amethyst** on the third eye (the area between the eyebrows) can enhance intuition, while placing **citrine** over the solar plexus chakra can stimulate personal power and will. **Clear quartz** can be placed over any chakra to amplify energy flow and promote balance.

- **Root Chakra**: Use grounding stones like **hematite** or **black tourmaline**.
- **Sacral Chakra**: **Carnelian** or **orange calcite** can stimulate creativity and passion.
- **Solar Plexus Chakra**: **Citrine** or **yellow jasper** can enhance personal power and confidence.
- **Heart Chakra**: **Rose quartz** or **green aventurine** can promote emotional healing and compassion.
- **Throat Chakra**: **Blue lace agate** or **lapis lazuli** can enhance communication and self-expression.
- **Third Eye Chakra**: **Amethyst** or **sodalite** can stimulate intuition and inner wisdom.
- **Crown Chakra**: **Clear quartz** or **selenite** can open the connection to higher consciousness.

Crystal Grid Meditation

For those seeking more advanced practices, creating a crystal grid around you can enhance the energy flow during meditation. Crystal grids involve placing multiple crystals in specific geometric patterns, often aligned to the body's energy centers or chakra system. This layout helps to amplify the energy of the crystals and direct it toward specific intentions. As you sit or lie in the center of the grid, the stones create a powerful energetic field that supports the meditation process, helping you to connect with your higher self or manifest specific intentions.

3. Enhancing Focus with Crystals

One of the key benefits of using crystals during meditation is their ability to enhance focus and concentration. Many people find that their minds tend to wander during meditation, making it difficult to achieve a deep meditative state. Crystals can help ground and stabilize your energy, making it easier to stay focused and present. For example, **smoky quartz** is known for its grounding properties, while **lapis lazuli** is excellent for enhancing mental clarity.

- **Hematite** is especially useful for grounding and can help you stay focused during meditation.
- **Fluorite** is known for clearing mental fog and enhancing concentration, making it ideal for meditation practices that require sharp focus or problem-solving.

4. Deepening Spiritual Connection

For those using meditation to deepen their spiritual connection or explore higher states of consciousness, crystals can act as a bridge between the physical and spiritual realms. **Clear quartz, amethyst,** and **selenite** are excellent for opening the crown chakra and connecting with divine energy. By focusing on these stones during meditation, you may experience heightened spiritual awareness, intuitive insights, or deeper states of consciousness.

- **Selenite** is often used to cleanse the aura and open up channels for spiritual guidance.
- **Labradorite** enhances connection to the spiritual realm, aiding in the exploration of higher consciousness.
- **Kyanite** can help align the chakras and create a harmonious flow of energy throughout the body.

5. Using Crystals for Manifestation

Crystals can also be incredibly powerful tools for manifestation meditation. By combining crystal energy with focused intention, you can manifest your desires more effectively. **Citrine,** known for attracting abundance, is ideal for manifesting financial success or personal goals. **Rose quartz** can be used in manifestation practices aimed at love, while **green aventurine** is often used to attract opportunities and good fortune.

To perform a manifestation meditation with crystals:

- Hold or place the crystal related to your intention (e.g., **citrine** for wealth, **rose quartz** for love) on your heart or crown chakra.
- Close your eyes, take deep breaths, and focus on your desired outcome.
- Visualize your intention coming to fruition, and allow the energy of the crystal to amplify your thoughts and desires.

6. Clearing and Balancing Energy

Crystals can also be used to clear and balance your energy field before, during, or after meditation. **Selenite** is one of the most powerful stones for energy clearing. It has a high vibrational frequency that can quickly remove negative energy and restore balance. Similarly, **black tourmaline** is used to absorb and transmute negative energies, creating a protective shield around you.

To clear and balance your energy:

- Use **selenite** or **clear quartz** to cleanse your aura before meditating.
- Place **black tourmaline** or **obsidian** at the corners of the room or near your body to absorb any negative energy and keep the space energetically clear.

7. The Power of Intention

The effectiveness of using crystals in meditation comes not only from the crystals themselves but from the intention you set during the process. Before you begin, take a moment to set a clear intention for your meditation—whether it's healing, relaxation, clarity, or spiritual growth. Hold this intention in your mind as you meditate with the crystals. The crystals will amplify and support your intention, helping you stay focused and aligned with your goals.

Conclusion

Meditation combined with crystals creates a potent practice for healing, clarity, spiritual growth, and manifestation. By choosing the right crystals for your specific needs and using them in creative and intentional ways, you can enhance your meditation practice and deepen your connection to your inner self and the universe. Whether you are seeking emotional balance, mental clarity, or spiritual enlightenment, crystals can act as powerful tools that elevate your meditation experience, bringing more focus, peace, and insight into your life.

Introduction to Crystal Meditation

Crystal meditation combines the ancient practice of meditation with the healing power of crystals. Crystals, with their unique vibrational frequencies, are thought to interact with the energy fields of the body to promote balance, healing, and alignment. By incorporating crystals into your meditation practice, you can deepen your connection to your inner self, enhance focus, and bring clarity to your mind. The energy of the crystals can support your intentions, whether for emotional healing, spiritual growth, or manifesting desires.

Each crystal possesses a distinct energy that can influence the chakras, meridians, and aura in specific ways. For example, **amethyst** is often used to promote calmness and spiritual awareness, while **rose quartz** is associated with emotional healing and self-love. **Clear quartz**, known as the "master healer," amplifies energy and intention, making it a versatile tool for any type of meditation.

During crystal meditation, the practitioner focuses on the energy of the crystal, allowing it to support and guide their meditation process. Whether holding a crystal in your hand, placing it on the body, or surrounding yourself with them, the crystals' vibrations can help clear mental clutter, facilitate deep relaxation, and open the mind to higher levels of consciousness. By aligning your intentions with the natural energies of the stones, you can enhance the effectiveness of your meditation practice and achieve more profound healing and insight.

Crystal meditation can be used to address specific issues such as stress, anxiety, or emotional blockages, or simply to deepen your spiritual practice and connection to the universe. Whether you're a beginner or experienced meditator, using crystals can serve as a valuable tool to enhance your journey toward balance and well-being.

Techniques for Meditating with Crystals

Meditating with crystals is a simple yet powerful way to enhance your practice and deepen your connection to the energy around you. By using the unique properties of crystals, you can create a focused, energetic environment that supports your physical, emotional, and spiritual well-being. Different techniques for meditating with crystals can help you harness their specific healing properties, whether you're looking for stress relief, emotional healing, or spiritual enlightenment. Here are several methods for integrating crystals into your meditation practice:

1. Holding Crystals During Meditation

One of the easiest and most accessible techniques is to hold a crystal in your hands while meditating. This method allows you to directly channel the crystal's energy into your body. Choose a crystal that resonates with your intention for the session. For example, holding **amethyst** can promote a calm, peaceful state, while **citrine** is excellent for boosting confidence and manifesting goals. Simply sit in a comfortable position, close your eyes, and focus on the sensations you feel from the crystal. Notice any subtle warmth, tingling, or vibrations that occur, and allow them to guide you deeper into a relaxed state.

2. Placing Crystals on the Body

Placing crystals on specific parts of your body, particularly the chakras, can help channel their energy directly to areas in need of healing. Each crystal corresponds with particular energy centers, and when placed on the body during meditation, it can facilitate energy flow and help restore balance.

For example:

- **Amethyst** on the third eye (between the eyebrows) enhances intuition and spiritual awareness.
- **Rose quartz** over the heart chakra promotes emotional healing and self-love.
- **Citrine** on the solar plexus can activate personal power and confidence.

While meditating, allow yourself to focus on the energy emanating from the crystals as you breathe deeply and relax. Pay attention to any shifts in energy, emotions, or physical sensations, and let the crystals guide you through the process.

3. Crystal Grids

A more advanced method of meditating with crystals is the use of a crystal grid. This technique involves arranging multiple crystals in a specific geometric pattern to amplify their energies. You can create a grid around your body, on your meditation space, or around a specific area where you want to manifest energy or intentions.

The pattern of the grid is essential, as certain shapes—such as circles, triangles, and squares—can direct and focus the energy in different ways. For example:

- **A circular grid** can help promote harmony and balance.
- **A triangular grid** can be used to boost creativity or enhance spiritual awakening.
- **A square grid** can create stability and grounding.

To enhance the grid's effectiveness, place a **clear quartz** crystal in the center, as it amplifies the energy of the surrounding stones. While meditating, sit in the center of the grid and focus on your intention, allowing the energy from the crystals to flow through you and into your surroundings.

4. Crystal Elixirs

Another popular technique for using crystals during meditation is to create a crystal elixir. This method involves placing a crystal in water (make sure it's safe to do so, as some stones are not water-safe) and letting the water absorb its energy. You can drink this water before or during meditation, allowing the crystal's energy to flow into your body as you meditate. Some people also use the water to cleanse the space or their aura before beginning their meditation session.

Note: Only use crystals that are safe for elixirs, such as **clear quartz**, **rose quartz**, or **amethyst**. Avoid stones like **malachite** or **sodalite**, which may be toxic when placed in water.

5. Chakra Balancing with Crystals

Chakra meditation with crystals is a powerful method for aligning the energy centers of the body. Each chakra is associated with a different color and energy frequency, and specific crystals resonate with each one. Placing the appropriate crystals on or near the corresponding chakra points can help balance and align your energy. Here's a quick guide to common crystals for chakra meditation:

- **Root Chakra (Muladhara): Hematite, black tourmaline**, or **red jasper**—used for grounding and stability.
- **Sacral Chakra (Svadhisthana): Carnelian, orange calcite**, or **moonstone**—for creativity and emotional balance.
- **Solar Plexus Chakra (Manipura): Citrine, yellow jasper**, or **amber**—for personal power and confidence.
- **Heart Chakra (Anahata): Rose quartz, green aventurine**, or **jade**—for love and compassion.
- **Throat Chakra (Vishuddha): Lapis lazuli, turquoise**, or **blue lace agate**—for clear communication.
- **Third Eye Chakra (Ajna): Amethyst, sodalite**, or **lapis lazuli**—for intuition and wisdom.
- **Crown Chakra (Sahasrara): Clear quartz, selenite**, or **diamond**—for spiritual connection and enlightenment.

During your meditation, visualize each chakra glowing with the corresponding color and energy as you place the crystals on or near those areas. This helps stimulate energy flow and restore balance to your body and mind.

6. Meditating with Crystals in Nature

If possible, meditating outdoors with crystals can amplify their grounding and healing effects. Crystals, especially those connected to the Earth, resonate well with natural surroundings. Find a quiet, peaceful spot in nature, such as a park, forest, or near water, and place your chosen crystals on the ground or around you. As you meditate, breathe in the natural energy and allow the crystals to connect with the Earth's vibrational frequencies, deepening your sense of grounding and connection.

7. Visualization and Intention Setting

During your meditation, it's important to focus on your intention for the session. Whether you are meditating for stress relief, healing, spiritual growth, or manifestation, keep your intention clear in your mind. Hold the crystal and visualize its energy merging with yours, expanding throughout your body or surrounding environment. Imagine your intention coming to life, supported and amplified by the crystal's vibrations.

For example, if you're using **citrine** for manifestation, visualize a bright, golden light growing within you, radiating outward and attracting opportunities and success. As you hold the crystal, keep your focus on your goal, allowing the energy to flow with purpose and clarity.

8. Sound and Crystal Meditation

Combining sound with crystal meditation can enhance the vibrational frequencies of both. Using sound healing instruments such as singing bowls, tuning forks, or even chanting can help you achieve a deeper state of meditation while amplifying the effects of the crystals. Place your crystals near the sound source or hold them while the sound vibrations fill the space, helping to open and balance your chakras. The resonance of the sound waves and the crystal energy work synergistically, enhancing the healing process.

Conclusion

Incorporating crystals into your meditation practice is an effective way to amplify your intentions, restore balance, and deepen your connection to yourself and the world around you. Whether you're holding crystals, placing them on your body, creating grids, or combining them with other techniques like sound, there are endless ways to experiment and enhance your practice. The key is to remain open to the experience, trust in the crystals' energy, and allow the healing process to unfold naturally.

Benefits of Crystal Meditation

Meditating with crystals offers a wide range of benefits, making it a valuable practice for anyone seeking emotional, physical, or spiritual healing. The unique energy vibrations of crystals are thought to interact with the body's energy field, clearing blockages, balancing the chakras, and promoting overall well-being. When combined with meditation, these benefits are amplified, creating a deeper, more focused experience that supports mental clarity, emotional stability, and spiritual growth.

1. Enhancing Emotional Healing

Crystals are often used to support emotional healing during meditation. Stones like **rose quartz** and **amethyst** can help to release negative emotions such as fear, anger, or grief. By holding or placing these stones on the body during meditation, individuals can connect with their heart chakra and encourage the release of emotional wounds. This can lead to greater emotional balance, increased self-love, and a stronger sense of inner peace. Rose quartz, for instance, is widely known for its ability to promote self-compassion and foster love in relationships, both with oneself and others.

2. Promoting Deep Relaxation

One of the most immediate benefits of crystal meditation is deep relaxation. Crystals such as **amethyst**, **blue lace agate**, and **sodalite** have calming properties that can help reduce stress and anxiety. As you meditate with these stones, their soothing energies promote a state of calm, allowing the body to release tension and the mind to quieten. Regular practice can result in reduced levels of cortisol (the stress hormone), enhanced relaxation, and better overall mental health. Crystals also have a way of grounding the practitioner, helping to anchor them in the present moment and dissolve feelings of overwhelm.

3. Boosting Mental Clarity and Focus

Crystals such as **clear quartz**, **fluorite**, and **tiger's eye** can help to improve mental clarity and focus during meditation. Clear quartz, for example, is known as the "master healer" because it amplifies energy and enhances clarity. When used during meditation, it can help clear the mind of mental fog, increase concentration, and bring greater focus to your intentions. Fluorite is often used for its ability to cleanse and stabilize the mind, making it easier to stay present and clear-headed during meditation. This is especially beneficial for those looking to work through mental blockages or seeking solutions to complex issues.

4. Stimulating Spiritual Growth

Crystal meditation can be a powerful tool for those seeking to deepen their spiritual practice or connect with higher consciousness. Stones like **amethyst, selenite, and lapis lazuli** are often used to stimulate the third eye and crown chakras, encouraging intuition, spiritual awakening, and connection to higher realms. Amethyst, in particular, is revered for its ability to enhance spiritual awareness and help individuals access higher states of consciousness. These crystals can guide you in your journey of self-discovery, meditation, and personal transformation, supporting your spiritual growth in profound ways.

5. Balancing and Aligning the Chakras

Crystals are known to correspond with specific chakras, and using them during meditation can help balance and align the energy centers of the body. By placing crystals on or near the body's chakra points, you can support the flow of energy, clear blockages, and restore harmony. For example, **green aventurine** is often used to balance the heart chakra, while **citrine** supports the solar plexus chakra, which governs personal power. By regularly meditating with crystals that align with the chakras, you can achieve a more balanced and harmonious state of being.

6. Manifesting Desires and Intentions

Crystals are powerful allies in the manifestation process. When used in meditation, they can amplify your intentions, helping you manifest your desires with greater ease. **Citrine** is particularly effective for attracting abundance and success, while **jade** is often used for prosperity and good fortune. During meditation, you can hold the crystal and focus on your intention, visualizing it coming to fruition. The energy of the crystal works in tandem with your focused thoughts and emotions to help bring your goals into reality. This synergy can create a stronger energetic alignment between your desires and the universe.

7. Clearing Negative Energy

Many crystals, especially **black tourmaline, smoky quartz**, and **selenite**, are known for their ability to clear negative energy. Whether you're working through emotional baggage or simply want to cleanse your environment, crystal meditation can help you clear away stagnant or harmful energies. Black tourmaline is often used to absorb and transmute negative energy, while selenite is a powerful cleanser that purifies the aura and the surrounding space. By meditating with these stones, you can create a healing space that encourages positivity and growth, free from the weight of negative emotions or external influences.

8. Improving Sleep Quality

Many people turn to crystal meditation as a way to improve their sleep quality. Crystals like **amethyst, howlite**, and **lepidolite** have calming and sedative effects that can help quiet the mind and prepare the body for restful sleep. By meditating with these stones before bed, you can promote a peaceful state of mind, reduce stress, and create a sense of tranquility that supports a good night's sleep. Howlite, in particular, is known for its ability to relieve anxiety and promote deep, restorative rest.

9. Increasing Self-Awareness

Crystal meditation can enhance self-awareness by helping you connect with your inner thoughts, emotions, and desires. As you meditate with crystals, especially those that support the heart or third eye chakras, you may gain deeper insights into your patterns, behaviors, and motivations. Crystals like **lapis lazuli** and **turquoise** encourage introspection and self-reflection, allowing you to gain clarity on areas of your life that need attention or healing. By cultivating a deeper understanding of yourself, you can make more conscious choices and live a more authentic life.

10. Strengthening Intuition and Psychic Abilities

Many practitioners use crystal meditation to strengthen their intuitive abilities and psychic gifts. Crystals like **amethyst, moonstone**, and **labradorite** are known for their ability to enhance intuition and open channels of communication with the spiritual realm. By meditating with these stones, you can develop a stronger sense of inner knowing, trust your instincts more fully, and gain greater clarity about your spiritual path. These crystals are often used to deepen psychic abilities such as clairvoyance, clairaudience, and other forms of extrasensory perception.

Conclusion

The benefits of crystal meditation are wide-ranging and deeply transformative. Whether you are seeking emotional healing, mental clarity, spiritual growth, or physical well-being, crystals can be powerful tools that support your journey. By incorporating crystals into your meditation practice, you can amplify your intentions, clear energetic blockages, and create a more balanced and harmonious life. Regular practice of crystal meditation can lead to lasting changes in how you feel, think, and relate to the world around you, offering both immediate relief and long-term benefits.

Crystal Healing for Emotional Balance

Crystals have long been used for their potential to promote emotional balance, offering a natural and holistic way to support mental and emotional well-being. The idea behind crystal healing for emotional balance is that the unique vibrations and energies emitted by certain stones can interact with the body's own energy field, helping to clear emotional blockages and restore harmony. By using specific crystals, you can address a wide range of emotional challenges such as stress, anxiety, grief, and depression, and foster a more positive emotional state.

1. Rose Quartz: The Stone of Love and Compassion

Known as the "stone of unconditional love," **rose quartz** is one of the most powerful crystals for emotional healing. It is often used to heal emotional wounds, especially those related to heartbreak, trauma, and self-love. Rose quartz promotes feelings of compassion, empathy, and kindness, both towards oneself and others. It can help open the heart chakra, encouraging emotional healing by dissolving negative emotions like anger, resentment, or guilt. Meditating with rose quartz or placing it on the heart chakra can foster self-acceptance, emotional balance, and an enhanced ability to give and receive love.

2. Amethyst: Calm and Clarity

Amethyst is a powerful crystal for promoting emotional peace and mental clarity. It is especially helpful for individuals experiencing stress, anxiety, or emotional overwhelm. Amethyst is known for its calming properties, helping to alleviate feelings of fear and nervous tension. It also supports the mind in clearing mental fog, promoting clearer thinking and decision-making. Meditating with amethyst can bring a sense of emotional stability, easing emotional turbulence and encouraging inner peace. It also helps with spiritual growth, providing protection against negative emotions and thoughts.

3. Citrine: Uplifting Energy

Often referred to as the "stone of joy," **citrine** is known for its ability to boost energy and promote a positive emotional state. It is particularly effective for overcoming feelings of depression, self-doubt, and negativity. Citrine's vibrant yellow energy is associated with the solar plexus chakra, which governs personal power, confidence, and self-esteem. When used in meditation or placed on the body, citrine can help release feelings of inadequacy, transforming them into self-confidence and optimism. It also supports manifestation, helping to manifest abundance and opportunities in life.

4. Lepidolite: Calming and Soothing

Lepidolite is often used to relieve stress, anxiety, and emotional imbalances. This stone contains **lithium**, a substance commonly used in psychiatric medicine to treat mood disorders, which is why it is believed to have a powerful calming effect on the emotional body. Lepidolite helps to bring emotional stability, particularly during times of transition, change, or personal crisis. It can ease feelings of depression, anxiety, and fear, helping to promote a more peaceful and balanced emotional state. Holding or meditating with lepidolite can support emotional healing and encourage mental clarity during difficult times.

5. Carnelian: Overcoming Fear and Anxiety

Carnelian is a warm, vibrant stone that is especially effective in helping individuals overcome fear, anxiety, and self-doubt. It is known for its ability to stimulate the root and sacral chakras, which are responsible for grounding, security, and emotional well-being. Carnelian can boost energy levels and improve motivation, making it ideal for individuals who feel stuck or unable to take action. It is particularly helpful for those recovering from emotional trauma, as it encourages emotional resilience and helps release feelings of anger, frustration, or sadness. Meditating with carnelian can bring emotional strength and clarity, helping to reignite passion and creativity.

6. Black Tourmaline: Protection from Negative Emotions

Black tourmaline is a powerful protective stone that can help shield against negative energy, including emotional toxicity from others. It is particularly beneficial for individuals who struggle with emotional overwhelm, as it can absorb and transmute negative emotions such as fear, anxiety, and anger. Black tourmaline helps to create a protective energy field around the user, guarding against external emotional influences that may be affecting their mental well-being. It is often used in combination with other crystals to provide an added layer of emotional security, especially during stressful or challenging situations.

7. Smoky Quartz: Grounding and Releasing Negative Energy

Smoky quartz is a grounding crystal that is highly effective for clearing negative energy, including emotional baggage. It is especially helpful for releasing feelings of sadness, depression, and grief. Smoky quartz works by absorbing and neutralizing negative energy, transforming it into positive vibrations. It also helps with emotional grounding, allowing individuals to stay balanced and centered during emotional upheaval. By meditating with smoky quartz, you can clear emotional blockages and restore emotional harmony. This crystal is particularly useful for those going through significant emotional transitions or facing long-term emotional challenges.

8. Fluorite: Emotional Healing and Clarity

Fluorite is known for its ability to clear negative energies and bring emotional clarity. This crystal is especially effective in helping individuals gain perspective during emotional confusion or turmoil. Fluorite works by clearing out mental clutter and emotional blockages, allowing the user to gain a clearer understanding of their emotional state and the root causes of their feelings. It is often used to help release negative emotional patterns, promote self-awareness, and foster mental clarity. Fluorite can also help balance the emotions, calming excessive emotional reactions and fostering a sense of calm and inner peace.

9. Turquoise: Healing and Communication

Turquoise is a stone that promotes emotional healing and enhances communication. It is particularly beneficial for individuals who struggle to express their emotions or communicate effectively with others. Turquoise encourages emotional balance by helping to release repressed emotions, providing a sense of freedom and release. It also facilitates clear communication, allowing individuals to express their feelings honestly and openly. Meditating with turquoise can help heal emotional wounds related to communication breakdowns, miscommunication, or emotional blockages, fostering healthier relationships and better self-expression.

10. Sodalite: Enhancing Intuition and Emotional Insight

Sodalite is a stone that enhances emotional insight, helping individuals gain clarity on their emotional needs and desires. It is particularly effective for those who experience emotional confusion or have difficulty understanding their feelings. Sodalite promotes introspection and self-awareness, making it easier to navigate complex emotions and gain a deeper understanding of their sources. This crystal also supports the throat chakra, enhancing communication and the ability to express emotions clearly. By meditating with sodalite, you can gain greater emotional clarity and access intuitive guidance for emotional healing.

Conclusion

Using crystals for emotional balance provides a holistic approach to emotional well-being, offering support and healing on an energetic level. By choosing the right crystals for your emotional needs, you can tap into their unique healing properties and restore harmony to your emotional body. Whether you are seeking relief from stress, anxiety, grief, or emotional blockages, crystals can offer a gentle, natural solution for finding balance, peace, and emotional resilience. Through regular meditation and mindful crystal use, you can create a more balanced emotional life, promoting healing, clarity, and a deep sense of inner calm.

Crystals for Peace and Tranquility

Crystals have been used for centuries to promote peace and tranquility, harnessing their natural energies to create a sense of calm and serenity in our lives. Each crystal carries its unique vibrational frequency, which can influence the energy around us and help to soothe the mind, body, and spirit. Whether you're seeking to reduce stress, calm anxiety, or foster a peaceful environment, certain crystals are particularly effective in promoting a deep sense of peace and tranquility.

1. Amethyst: Calming the Mind

Amethyst is widely regarded as one of the most effective crystals for peace and relaxation. Its calming energy helps to alleviate stress and mental tension, promoting clarity and inner peace. This crystal is known for its ability to calm the mind and balance the emotions, making it an ideal companion for those experiencing anxiety or emotional overwhelm. Amethyst also supports the third eye and crown chakras, enhancing spiritual awareness and helping individuals to access higher states of consciousness. Meditating with amethyst can create a peaceful mental space, making it easier to let go of negative thoughts and emotions.

2. Sodalite: Peace through Communication

Sodalite is a crystal that encourages emotional balance and peaceful communication. It is particularly effective for calming the mind and releasing negative thought patterns that may cause mental and emotional unrest. Sodalite works by clearing mental fog, allowing for greater clarity and understanding. This stone also promotes the healthy expression of emotions and thoughts, making it useful for those who find it difficult to express themselves or communicate their feelings. By promoting emotional honesty and openness, sodalite creates an atmosphere of peace, both within oneself and in relationships.

3. Rose Quartz: Nurturing Love and Calm

Rose quartz, known as the stone of unconditional love, is a powerful crystal for fostering peace and tranquility in relationships. It helps to open the heart chakra and encourages self-love, compassion, and emotional healing. When used for meditation or placed in a room, rose quartz can reduce stress and anxiety, bringing a gentle sense of calm and comfort. It is particularly effective in soothing emotional wounds, helping to release feelings of grief, anger, or resentment. By promoting feelings of love and understanding, rose quartz encourages peaceful interactions and creates a serene environment.

4. Lepidolite: Calm and Soothing Energy

Lepidolite is known for its calming and soothing properties, making it an excellent choice for those seeking to alleviate stress, anxiety, and emotional turmoil. This crystal contains lithium, which is often used in treatments for mood disorders, and is particularly effective for stabilizing emotions. Lepidolite helps to balance the mind and body, encouraging a sense of relaxation and peace. It also aids in releasing negative thought patterns and emotional blockages, allowing for a greater flow of positive energy. Meditating with lepidolite can promote emotional healing and restore a sense of inner peace.

5. Black Tourmaline: Grounding and Protection

Black tourmaline is a grounding crystal that offers protection from negative energies, making it a valuable tool for creating a peaceful and harmonious environment. This stone is known for its ability to absorb and transmute negative energy, including emotional stress and anxiety. It helps to clear the energy field, promoting a sense of calm and security. By grounding the user in the present moment, black tourmaline helps to alleviate feelings of restlessness and unease. Placing black tourmaline in the home or workspace can help create a peaceful, balanced atmosphere, free from negative emotional influences.

6. Celestite: Soothing the Soul

Celestite is a crystal known for its gentle, calming energy. It is often used to promote inner peace, relaxation, and tranquility. This stone connects with the higher realms and encourages spiritual growth, making it a wonderful tool for those seeking to deepen their spiritual practice. Celestite's soft blue energy is associated with the throat and third eye chakras, encouraging clear communication and a peaceful mind. When used for meditation, celestite helps to ease mental tension and promote a serene, meditative state, allowing for a deeper sense of peace and spiritual connection.

7. Howlite: Tranquility and Patience

Howlite is a soothing crystal that promotes tranquility and patience. It is often used to calm the mind and reduce stress, making it a helpful tool for those experiencing frustration or agitation. Howlite's gentle energy encourages emotional balance and self-reflection, helping individuals to release negative thoughts and feelings. This stone is also known for its ability to foster patience and understanding, particularly in challenging situations. Meditating with howlite can create a peaceful state of mind, allowing for a greater sense of emotional calm and inner stillness.

8. Aquamarine: Gentle Calm and Clarity

Aquamarine is a crystal that promotes gentle calmness and emotional clarity. It is particularly effective for soothing nervous tension and reducing feelings of anxiety or overwhelm. Aquamarine's calming energy is associated with the throat chakra, supporting clear communication and self-expression. This stone encourages emotional healing by helping individuals release fear and negative emotions, promoting peace and tranquility in both the mind and body. Aquamarine is also known for its ability to bring clarity during difficult emotional situations, helping to reduce mental confusion and promote peaceful resolution.

9. Green Aventurine: Relaxation and Harmony

Green aventurine is a crystal that encourages relaxation and emotional harmony. Known for its calming green energy, this stone is often used to promote balance and peacefulness, particularly in times of stress or emotional upheaval. Green aventurine works by clearing blockages in the heart chakra, helping to release negative emotions such as anger, jealousy, or frustration. It also supports emotional healing by promoting a sense of abundance, luck, and well-being. Meditating with green aventurine can help create a harmonious emotional state, fostering a sense of peace and relaxation.

10. Chrysoprase: Emotional Healing and Calm

Chrysoprase is a crystal that promotes emotional healing and inner calm. It helps to release negative emotions and brings peace to the heart and mind. Chrysoprase is known for its ability to open the heart chakra, encouraging the flow of love, compassion, and understanding. This stone also promotes forgiveness, helping to release old emotional wounds and grievances. By fostering a sense of emotional balance, chrysoprase can create a more peaceful and serene environment, both within oneself and in relationships with others.

Conclusion

Crystals have long been valued for their ability to create a sense of peace and tranquility in our lives. By harnessing the unique energies of specific stones, we can foster emotional balance, reduce stress, and create a calming environment. Whether you're seeking to relieve anxiety, enhance spiritual growth, or promote harmonious relationships, crystals like amethyst, rose quartz, and lepidolite can offer the support you need. Through meditation, mindful use, or simply placing these stones in your environment, you can invite peace and tranquility into your life, cultivating a deeper sense of calm and serenity.

Crystals for Confidence and Self-Esteem

Crystals are powerful tools for boosting confidence and self-esteem, helping to empower individuals by harmonizing the body's energy fields. By tapping into the unique frequencies of certain stones, you can strengthen your sense of self-worth, overcome self-doubt, and unlock your full potential. Whether you're preparing for a public speaking event, seeking personal growth, or working through feelings of inadequacy, there are specific crystals that can support your journey toward self-confidence and greater self-love.

1. Citrine: The Stone of Personal Power

Citrine is a bright, energizing stone often referred to as the "success stone" or the "merchant's stone" because of its association with abundance and personal power. It's especially helpful for boosting confidence and self-esteem by encouraging a positive, can-do attitude. Citrine's vibrant energy works with the solar plexus chakra, which governs self-confidence, willpower, and personal strength. By wearing or meditating with citrine, you can increase your sense of empowerment, dispel negative thoughts, and replace them with optimism and determination. This stone fosters a sense of joy and vitality, helping to overcome feelings of inferiority and building a more positive self-image.

2. Tiger's Eye: Strength and Courage

Tiger's eye is a grounding and protective stone that enhances confidence and courage. It helps to eliminate fear and self-doubt while promoting clarity and focus. Associated with the root and solar plexus chakras, tiger's eye encourages emotional strength and stability. It is often used by individuals who need to take bold actions or make difficult decisions. Meditating with tiger's eye can provide the mental clarity needed to overcome uncertainty, while its grounding nature ensures that your confidence is rooted in a sense of reality, helping you to stay grounded even in challenging situations.

3. Carnelian: Creativity and Motivation

Carnelian is a vibrant orange stone that stimulates both creativity and motivation, while also enhancing self-esteem. It is known for its ability to activate the sacral and solar plexus chakras, which govern creativity, personal power, and self-worth. When you're feeling stuck or lacking in confidence, carnelian can reignite your passion and enthusiasm, encouraging you to take action and pursue your goals. This stone also helps you release feelings of fear or self-doubt that may be holding you back, enabling you to move forward with greater energy and self-assurance.

4. Rose Quartz: Love and Self-Acceptance

Though rose quartz is often associated with love and relationships, its gentle energy is also incredibly effective for fostering self-love and acceptance. This soft pink crystal works with the heart chakra to heal emotional wounds and encourage a deep sense of self-compassion. By meditating with rose quartz, you can release feelings of inadequacy or unworthiness and replace them with kindness and understanding toward yourself. It is especially helpful for those who struggle with negative self-talk or who feel disconnected from their own self-worth. Rose quartz fosters an open heart, allowing you to embrace yourself with love and acceptance, which is a key foundation for building true confidence.

5. Clear Quartz: Amplifying Personal Strength

Clear quartz is a versatile and powerful crystal that can amplify the energy of other stones, making it an excellent addition to any confidence-boosting practice. It is often used to enhance clarity of thought, mental focus, and personal power. Clear quartz works with all of the chakras, but it is particularly effective for the crown chakra, supporting the expansion of consciousness and spiritual clarity. Using clear quartz in meditation can help to clear any mental blocks that may be hindering your self-confidence and encourage a stronger connection to your higher self. It also amplifies your intention for success, helping to manifest your goals more effectively.

6. Lapis Lazuli: Wisdom and Inner Truth

Lapis lazuli is a stone of wisdom and self-expression. It stimulates the throat and third eye chakras, enhancing communication and inner truth. When you're trying to boost your confidence, particularly in expressing your true thoughts and feelings, lapis lazuli can help you speak with clarity and conviction. This stone encourages you to trust in your inner wisdom and intuition, reinforcing your sense of self-worth. Lapis lazuli also helps you to recognize and embrace your strengths, while dissolving any limiting beliefs or self-doubt that may be undermining your confidence.

7. Amazonite: Courage and Self-Expression

Amazonite is a stone of courage and self-expression, particularly when it comes to overcoming fears and self-imposed limitations. This turquoise-green crystal works with the heart and throat chakras, helping you to express your true emotions while also encouraging emotional balance. Amazonite helps to dispel negative energy and self-doubt, making it easier to speak up for yourself and stand in your personal power. Whether you're preparing for a difficult conversation or trying to assert yourself in challenging situations, amazonite can support you by fostering a greater sense of self-assurance and confidence.

8. Malachite: Transformation and Self-Discovery

Malachite is known for its transformative properties, helping to heal emotional wounds and facilitate personal growth. This powerful green crystal works with the heart chakra, clearing emotional blockages and encouraging a deeper connection to your authentic self. Malachite is particularly helpful when you're going through periods of change or personal development, as it helps to build resilience and self-reliance. It supports the process of self-discovery, allowing you to recognize your inherent strengths and abilities. As malachite helps to release old emotional patterns, it makes space for the growth of confidence and self-esteem.

9. Pyrite: Confidence and Manifestation

Often called "Fool's Gold," **pyrite** is a powerful crystal for manifesting wealth, success, and self-confidence. It stimulates the solar plexus chakra, promoting personal power, leadership, and the confidence to pursue your ambitions. Pyrite enhances your ability to take action toward your goals and encourages you to step into your full potential without hesitation. It also provides energetic protection, shielding you from negative influences and boosting your mental clarity. By meditating with pyrite, you can increase your confidence and take bold steps toward achieving your desires.

10. Sunstone: Joy and Optimism

Sunstone is a bright, radiant crystal that promotes joy, optimism, and personal power. It is associated with the sacral and solar plexus chakras, both of which influence self-esteem, vitality, and emotional expression. Sunstone helps to release feelings of guilt, shame, or unworthiness, replacing them with positive energy and enthusiasm for life. It encourages an open and confident expression of who you truly are, helping you to step into your own light and embrace your unique talents and qualities. Sunstone also encourages a sense of adventure and excitement, reminding you that you have the power to create the life you desire.

Conclusion

Crystals offer an accessible and natural way to enhance your confidence and self-esteem, providing support for personal growth and empowerment. Whether you choose the vibrant energy of citrine, the protective power of tiger's eye, or the soothing love of rose quartz, each crystal carries unique qualities that can help you strengthen your self-belief and unlock your potential. By incorporating these stones into your daily practice—whether through meditation, wearing crystal jewelry, or simply keeping them nearby—you can create a powerful energetic shift that supports your journey toward greater confidence and self-empowerment.

Crystals for Love and Relationships

Crystals have been used for centuries to enhance love, deepen relationships, and heal emotional wounds. Their natural energies can help to open the heart chakra, foster emotional balance, and attract positive energy into your relationships. Whether you're seeking to nurture existing connections, manifest new love, or heal past emotional scars, specific crystals can be powerful allies in your journey toward greater love and intimacy.

1. Rose Quartz: The Stone of Unconditional Love

Rose quartz is perhaps the most well-known crystal for love, earning its reputation as the stone of unconditional love and compassion. Its gentle pink energy works to heal emotional wounds, open the heart chakra, and encourage self-love, which is essential for attracting and maintaining healthy relationships. Rose quartz helps to dissolve feelings of resentment, anger, or heartbreak, allowing for forgiveness and emotional healing. It also promotes harmony in relationships by encouraging mutual understanding, compassion, and unconditional love. Keeping rose quartz in your home or wearing it as jewelry can create a loving, peaceful environment, attracting positive energy into your relationships.

2. Rhodochrosite: Compassion and Emotional Healing

Rhodochrosite is a powerful crystal for emotional healing and compassion. Known for its deep pink and red hues, this stone works to heal the heart chakra and restore balance to your emotions. Rhodochrosite is particularly helpful for individuals who have experienced emotional trauma, heartbreak, or rejection. It encourages self-acceptance and compassion, allowing you to release old emotional wounds and create space for healthier, more loving relationships. Rhodochrosite also helps to strengthen the bonds between partners by fostering mutual understanding, empathy, and emotional connection.

3. Carnelian: Passion and Vitality

Carnelian is an energizing and vibrant crystal that stimulates the sacral chakra, the center of creativity, sexuality, and passion. This stone helps to reignite the passion and vitality in romantic relationships, making it an excellent choice for couples looking to reconnect or enhance intimacy. Carnelian encourages emotional openness, self-expression, and courage, making it easier to share your feelings and desires with your partner. It can also help you to attract new love by boosting your confidence and allowing you to express yourself authentically. As a stone of creativity, carnelian can also inspire fresh ideas and approaches to enhancing your relationship.

4. Amethyst: Peace and Spiritual Connection

Amethyst, a stone of spiritual growth and inner peace, works with the crown and third eye chakras to deepen spiritual connections between partners. It encourages mutual respect, understanding, and trust, which are key ingredients for long-lasting, harmonious relationships. Amethyst helps to alleviate stress, anxiety, and emotional turbulence, allowing for clearer communication and more meaningful interactions. This crystal also aids in resolving conflicts by promoting calmness and emotional clarity. Amethyst is particularly useful for couples seeking to create a peaceful, balanced relationship that is grounded in love and mutual respect.

5. Garnet: Passion and Commitment

Garnet is a stone that promotes passion, commitment, and stability in relationships. This deep red crystal works with the root and sacral chakras, enhancing both physical and emotional intimacy. Garnet fosters loyalty and commitment, helping partners to strengthen their bond and maintain a deep emotional connection. It also promotes sensuality and desire, making it an excellent stone for reigniting the spark in long-term relationships. Garnet encourages honest communication, mutual support, and a deep sense of connection, ensuring that the relationship remains passionate, grounded, and fulfilling.

6. Lapis Lazuli: Truth and Communication

Lapis lazuli is a powerful crystal for enhancing communication and fostering honesty in relationships. Known for its rich blue color, it works with the throat chakra, helping individuals to speak their truth and express their feelings openly. Lapis lazuli encourages clear, direct communication, which is essential for resolving conflicts and deepening trust in relationships. It also helps to enhance emotional intelligence, allowing you to better understand your partner's needs and feelings. By promoting authentic self-expression, lapis lazuli can help to create a more open, transparent, and harmonious dynamic between partners.

7. Turquoise: Healing and Harmony

Turquoise is a healing stone that promotes harmony, balance, and emotional healing within relationships. It works with the throat chakra to enhance communication and encourages emotional expression in a gentle, non-confrontational way. Turquoise is particularly useful for couples who may be going through difficult times or who struggle to communicate effectively. This crystal helps to open the heart and mind, fostering understanding and empathy between partners. It also aids in overcoming past emotional wounds, making it an excellent choice for healing from past relationships and creating space for new love to grow.

8. Clear Quartz: Amplification and Clarity

Clear quartz is a versatile crystal that can be used to amplify the energy of other stones, making it an excellent addition to any crystal healing practice for love. It works with all of the chakras and helps to clear blockages, promoting emotional balance and clarity in relationships. Clear quartz encourages open, honest communication and helps to amplify the positive energies of love, trust, and understanding. By wearing or meditating with clear quartz, you can gain greater clarity about your relationship needs and desires, as well as create a deeper connection with your partner.

9. Moonstone: Intuition and Emotional Balance

Moonstone is a crystal that enhances intuition, emotional balance, and empathy, making it an excellent stone for deepening relationships. Its soft, feminine energy works with the crown and third eye chakras, allowing you to trust your inner wisdom and gain insight into the emotional needs of yourself and your partner. Moonstone helps to calm emotional turbulence, creating a peaceful and balanced atmosphere in relationships. It also supports new beginnings, making it a wonderful crystal for those seeking to attract new love or begin a fresh chapter in their current relationship.

10. Prehnite: Unconditional Love and Protection

Prehnite is a crystal that embodies unconditional love and emotional protection. It works with the heart chakra to nurture compassion and selflessness in relationships. Prehnite encourages healing and growth, allowing you to release emotional blockages and approach relationships with an open heart. This crystal also protects against negative energies, creating a safe and nurturing environment for love to flourish. Prehnite is ideal for those who want to strengthen their emotional bonds and build a relationship based on mutual respect, understanding, and unconditional love.

Conclusion

Crystals are valuable tools for enhancing love and relationships, providing both emotional healing and energetic support. Whether you're seeking to attract new love, heal from past wounds, or deepen your connection with a partner, there are crystals to support every stage of your journey. By working with stones such as rose quartz, rhodochrosite, and carnelian, you can cultivate an atmosphere of love, harmony, and mutual respect, creating space for healthier, more fulfilling relationships. The energy of crystals can help to align your heart, mind, and spirit, making it easier to connect with others on a deeper, more meaningful level

Crystal Healing for Physical Well-Being

Crystals have long been revered for their potential to enhance physical well-being by supporting the body's natural healing processes. While they are not a substitute for medical treatment, many people turn to crystals as a complementary approach to help manage physical ailments, promote overall vitality, and balance the body's energies. Crystals can work in a variety of ways, such as by stimulating circulation, reducing inflammation, boosting immunity, and easing pain. Through their energetic properties, they align with the body's subtle energy systems, including the chakras and meridians, to encourage balance and harmony.

1. Amethyst: Pain Relief and Stress Reduction

Amethyst is often used to alleviate physical pain, particularly headaches and migraines, due to its calming and soothing properties. This deep purple crystal is known for its ability to reduce stress and anxiety, which in turn can help ease tension-related discomfort. Amethyst's connection to the crown and third eye chakras enhances relaxation, helping the body to release pent-up stress that might be contributing to physical pain. Additionally, amethyst is said to assist in the regeneration of cells, making it beneficial for healing after injury or surgery. It is often placed on the forehead or temples to soothe headaches or worn as jewelry to maintain a calm, balanced energy throughout the day.

2. Clear Quartz: Energy Amplifier and Detoxifier

Clear quartz is one of the most versatile healing crystals, often referred to as the "master healer." Its primary function is to amplify the energy of other crystals, making it an excellent addition to any healing practice. When it comes to physical well-being, clear quartz is thought to support the body's detoxification processes by clearing negative energy and blockages. It helps to balance the energy flow through the body, which can improve circulation, enhance immunity, and promote overall vitality. Clear quartz is also used to enhance the body's natural ability to heal itself, making it ideal for use during recovery from illness or injury. It is often placed on the body or used in combination with other healing stones to facilitate energy flow and healing.

3. Hematite: Grounding and Circulation Support

Hematite is a grounding stone that is often used to improve circulation, increase energy, and support the body's natural detoxification systems. Its deep metallic sheen helps to draw excess heat away from the body, which can be beneficial for reducing inflammation and promoting better blood flow. Hematite is particularly helpful for conditions like varicose veins, poor circulation, or any issues related to blood flow. By grounding the body and stabilizing energy, hematite also helps reduce feelings of fatigue and enhances overall vitality. It is commonly worn as jewelry or carried as a pocket stone to keep the energy grounded and balanced throughout the day.

4. Carnelian: Boosting Energy and Vitality

Carnelian is a vibrant orange stone that is known for its ability to stimulate energy, vitality, and motivation. It is often used to promote physical strength and stamina, making it a great crystal for anyone recovering from illness or looking to enhance their overall physical well-being. Carnelian works by stimulating the root and sacral chakras, which are responsible for grounding energy and supporting physical vitality. It helps to energize the body, improve metabolism, and support the immune system. As an energizing crystal, carnelian can also help to overcome feelings of sluggishness or fatigue, making it ideal for those needing a boost in physical energy or motivation.

5. Turquoise: Healing and Detoxification

Turquoise is a stone known for its healing and detoxifying properties. It is often used to support the immune system and enhance the body's natural ability to heal itself. Turquoise is also considered beneficial for the respiratory system, helping to relieve conditions like coughs, asthma, or other respiratory issues. This crystal has a natural ability to cleanse and purify the body, making it especially useful in detoxification practices. Its calming and soothing properties can help reduce inflammation and ease pain in the joints, muscles, and other parts of the body. When placed on the body or worn as jewelry, turquoise promotes physical health by enhancing the body's energy flow and overall vitality.

6. Rose Quartz: Circulation and Heart Health

Rose quartz, known for its connection to love and compassion, also has powerful physical healing properties, particularly related to the heart and circulatory system. It is often used to support heart health by improving circulation, reducing stress, and promoting emotional healing. Rose quartz helps to open the heart chakra, encouraging love and self-care, which can have a direct impact on overall health. By relieving emotional stress and trauma, rose quartz helps to lower blood pressure and promote relaxation, which in turn benefits heart health. Its gentle energy encourages the body to relax and release any tension that could be negatively impacting the heart and circulatory system.

7. Black Tourmaline: Protection and Stress Relief

Black tourmaline is primarily known for its protective and grounding properties, but it also offers benefits for physical health by alleviating stress and promoting relaxation. When the body is under stress, it can manifest as physical symptoms, including headaches, muscle tension, and digestive issues. Black tourmaline is thought to absorb negative energy and block electromagnetic radiation, creating a protective barrier around the body. This helps to reduce stress levels and protect the body from harmful environmental influences. It is often used in healing practices to promote relaxation and support overall physical health, especially when dealing with the effects of stress or environmental toxicity.

8. Selenite: Healing and Cleansing

Selenite is a powerful crystal that is used to cleanse and recharge other crystals, but it is also highly beneficial for the body's physical well-being. Selenite's energy is thought to promote healing by removing blockages from the body's energetic pathways, allowing the natural healing process to take place. It is particularly helpful for conditions involving inflammation, muscle soreness, or any type of physical tension. Selenite also works to clear negative energies, which can have a direct impact on physical health by improving mental clarity and overall energy flow. It is often used during meditation or placed around the body to facilitate deep healing and restoration.

9. Malachite: Pain Relief and Detoxification

Malachite is known for its potent healing properties and is often used for its ability to relieve pain, reduce inflammation, and support detoxification. It is especially effective for conditions related to the joints, muscles, and bones, including arthritis, back pain, or muscle spasms. Malachite is thought to draw out negative energies from the body and clear blockages that may be hindering physical healing. Its energy helps to stimulate circulation, reduce swelling, and support the body's ability to regenerate tissues and cells. Malachite can be placed on areas of the body that are in pain, or it can be worn as jewelry for continuous support.

10. Chrysoprase: Immune System Support

Chrysoprase, a variety of chalcedony, is a stone that promotes healing and supports the immune system. It is thought to help the body recover from illness and prevent the recurrence of infection or disease. Chrysoprase works by promoting the detoxification of the body and enhancing energy flow. It is particularly beneficial for those who suffer from recurring illnesses, as it helps to strengthen the immune system and increase overall vitality. Chrysoprase also has a calming and balancing effect on the body, making it helpful for those dealing with chronic stress, which can negatively impact physical health.

Conclusion

Crystals can serve as powerful tools in supporting physical well-being, enhancing the body's natural healing abilities, and promoting overall vitality. Whether used to reduce pain, boost energy, support the immune system, or aid in detoxification, the right crystals can help create a balanced and harmonious energy field that supports your physical health. By working with stones like amethyst, carnelian, and turquoise, you can tap into their natural healing properties to improve your physical state and well-being.

Crystals for General Health and Wellness

Crystals have been valued for centuries not only for their aesthetic beauty but also for their purported ability to support health and wellness. Each type of crystal is thought to possess unique energy properties that resonate with the body's subtle energy systems, helping to restore balance and promote overall well-being. While crystal healing should not be seen as a replacement for medical treatment, many people incorporate crystals into their holistic wellness practices to improve physical, emotional, and spiritual health. Here are some popular crystals known for their positive impact on general health and wellness.

1. Clear Quartz: Master Healer and Energizer

Clear quartz is often referred to as the "master healer" because of its versatile healing properties. This transparent crystal is known to amplify the energy of other stones, making it a powerful ally in any crystal healing practice. It is thought to support the immune system, enhance energy flow, and promote general vitality. Clear quartz helps to cleanse the body of negative energies, reducing stress and bringing a sense of clarity and calm. Whether worn as jewelry, carried as a pocket stone, or placed around the home, clear quartz is believed to enhance overall health by stimulating the body's natural healing mechanisms.

2. Amethyst: Stress Relief and Sleep Aid

Amethyst, with its calming purple hues, is widely used to promote relaxation and alleviate stress. It is known for its ability to calm the mind, making it an excellent crystal for reducing anxiety and insomnia. Amethyst is also beneficial for supporting emotional balance, helping to clear negative thought patterns and encourage mental clarity. By working with the crown chakra, amethyst enhances spiritual awareness and supports a deeper sense of inner peace. Many people place amethyst under their pillow or by their bedside to promote restful sleep and alleviate tension or stress from the day.

3. Rose Quartz: Heart Healing and Emotional Wellness

Rose quartz is the crystal of unconditional love, making it an excellent tool for emotional healing. It is especially beneficial for those who are struggling with grief, heartbreak, or emotional wounds, as it helps to heal the heart chakra and release past trauma. Rose quartz encourages self-love, compassion, and forgiveness, which are key elements in maintaining emotional wellness. It also promotes peaceful relationships, both with others and with oneself, by fostering understanding, kindness, and empathy. Keeping rose quartz close, such as in your home or as a piece of jewelry, can create a soothing environment that nurtures emotional balance and healing.

4. Citrine: Joy and Vitality

Citrine is often associated with the energy of the sun, bringing warmth, joy, and vitality into one's life. This bright yellow crystal is known for its ability to uplift mood and promote positivity, making it a great stone for those experiencing feelings of depression or negativity. Citrine is believed to boost energy levels, support digestion, and stimulate mental clarity. As a stone of abundance, it is also thought to attract success and prosperity into one's life. By working with citrine, individuals can experience a greater sense of optimism and vitality, enhancing their overall wellness and well-being.

5. Black Tourmaline: Protection and Grounding

Black tourmaline is a protective stone that is often used to shield the body from negative energies and environmental toxins. It is known for its grounding qualities, helping to create a sense of stability and safety in times of stress or emotional turbulence. Black tourmaline is also thought to help detoxify the body by absorbing harmful energies, making it an excellent tool for those who are sensitive to electromagnetic fields (EMFs) from electronic devices. Carrying or wearing black tourmaline can create a protective energy field around the body, which promotes a sense of security and physical well-being.

6. Lapis Lazuli: Mental Clarity and Communication

Lapis lazuli is a deep blue stone that is known to enhance mental clarity and promote effective communication. It stimulates the third eye and throat chakras, allowing for better self-expression and a deeper understanding of one's own thoughts and feelings. Lapis lazuli is also believed to improve concentration and memory, making it useful for those seeking mental sharpness and focus. In terms of general wellness, lapis lazuli supports both emotional and physical healing by promoting inner peace, reducing stress, and encouraging personal growth.

7. Selenite: Purification and Energy Cleansing

Selenite is a crystal that is often used for cleansing and purification. It is known to have powerful energy-clearing properties, helping to remove negative or stagnant energies from the body, mind, and environment. Selenite is especially useful in creating a high-vibration atmosphere in your home or healing space. It is believed to help release physical blockages, relieve pain, and promote a sense of calm and well-being. Selenite can also be used to recharge other crystals, making it an essential part of any crystal healing toolkit. Placing selenite near your bed or in your living space is said to enhance the flow of positive energy and support overall health.

8. Fluorite: Mental and Physical Detox

Fluorite is known for its detoxifying properties, working to cleanse both the mind and body of harmful energies. It is often used to clear mental fog, improve concentration, and support intellectual decision-making. On a physical level, fluorite is believed to support the immune system and detoxify the body, helping to rid it of toxins and harmful substances. Fluorite is also used to balance the energy of the chakras, bringing clarity and harmony to both physical and emotional health. Its purifying energy helps to restore balance and vitality, making it an excellent crystal for maintaining overall wellness.

9. Carnelian: Motivation and Physical Energy

Carnelian is an energizing stone known for its ability to stimulate physical vitality, creativity, and motivation. This bright orange crystal works to activate the root and sacral chakras, which govern energy, action, and physical strength. Carnelian is commonly used to boost energy levels, improve circulation, and support overall physical vitality. It also helps to overcome feelings of sluggishness, fatigue, or lack of motivation, making it ideal for those seeking an energy boost or trying to get back on track with physical goals. By increasing confidence and enthusiasm, carnelian supports a more active and healthy lifestyle.

10. Green Aventurine: Prosperity and Healing

Green aventurine is often called the "stone of opportunity" because of its ability to attract good fortune and prosperity. It is also a powerful crystal for physical healing, particularly for the heart and cardiovascular system. Green aventurine is believed to stimulate healing processes in the body, support the immune system, and promote a general sense of well-being. It also aids in the release of negative energies and stress, making it easier for the body to achieve balance and vitality. Green aventurine is a great crystal for those looking to boost their health and wellness while manifesting success and positive energy in their lives.

11. Moonstone: Emotional Balance and Physical Harmony

Moonstone is a soothing stone that encourages emotional balance and harmony. Its gentle energy helps to stabilize mood swings, reduce stress, and promote restful sleep. Moonstone is often used for its ability to align the body's internal rhythms, supporting the endocrine and reproductive systems. It is also thought to promote physical healing by balancing the flow of energy throughout the body. Moonstone's connection to the feminine energy makes it especially useful for women's health, particularly in regulating menstrual cycles and supporting hormonal balance.

Conclusion

Crystals can serve as valuable tools in maintaining general health and wellness by supporting the body's natural healing abilities, promoting emotional balance, and enhancing mental clarity. Whether used for stress relief, detoxification, vitality, or protection, each crystal offers unique properties that contribute to overall well-being. Incorporating crystals into your daily routine—whether through meditation, wearing them as jewelry, or simply placing them in your environment—can create a harmonious energy that nurtures the body, mind, and spirit, ultimately promoting a healthier, more balanced life.

Crystals for Specific Physical Ailments

Crystals are often used in alternative healing practices to help alleviate specific physical ailments. While not a substitute for conventional medical treatment, many people turn to crystals as complementary tools to support the body's natural healing processes. Each crystal carries a unique energetic vibration that is believed to interact with the body's energy field, promoting healing and relieving physical discomfort. Whether used to alleviate pain, reduce inflammation, or improve circulation, these stones have been valued for their potential to address a wide range of physical health concerns.

1. Amethyst for Headaches and Migraines

Amethyst is often used to help soothe headaches and migraines, particularly those caused by stress or tension. Its calming properties can relieve mental and emotional stress, which are common triggers for headaches. Amethyst is believed to work by reducing the intensity of pain, improving blood circulation, and calming the nervous system. Placing amethyst on the forehead or temples can bring relief, as it is said to promote relaxation and alleviate tension in the head and neck. For chronic migraine sufferers, using amethyst during meditation or keeping the stone close may help manage symptoms.

2. Hematite for Circulation Issues and Blood Disorders

Hematite is known for its grounding and circulation-enhancing properties, making it particularly helpful for those with circulation problems or blood-related conditions. Hematite is believed to stimulate the flow of blood and oxygen throughout the body, which may support overall heart health. It is often used for conditions such as varicose veins, poor circulation, and anemia. By placing hematite on areas of the body that need attention or wearing it as jewelry, people can harness its energy to improve circulation and support the blood's natural function.

3. Rose Quartz for Heart Health and Blood Pressure

Rose quartz, often associated with love and compassion, also has physical healing properties, particularly for the heart and circulatory system. It is believed to improve circulation and regulate blood pressure by fostering emotional balance and reducing stress, which can contribute to heart-related issues. Rose quartz's gentle energy is said to calm the nervous system, lower blood pressure, and encourage self-care and healing. For those with heart conditions or high blood pressure, placing rose quartz over the heart or wearing it as jewelry may help maintain a sense of calm and emotional stability.

4. Turquoise for Respiratory and Immune System Support

Turquoise has long been regarded as a powerful healing stone for the respiratory system. It is thought to promote clear breathing by easing conditions such as asthma, bronchitis, and colds. Turquoise is believed to have detoxifying properties that help cleanse the body of toxins, supporting the immune system and improving overall health. Wearing turquoise or using it during meditation can help strengthen the immune system, reduce inflammation in the lungs, and promote respiratory wellness. It is also said to help with allergies by reducing their severity and improving overall vitality.

5. Carnelian for Fatigue and Digestive Issues

Carnelian is a vibrant orange crystal known for its energizing properties. It is often used to combat fatigue, increase vitality, and boost physical strength. Carnelian stimulates the root and sacral chakras, which are associated with energy, motivation, and vitality. This makes it an excellent stone for those feeling sluggish or lacking in energy, as it helps to invigorate the body and mind. In addition, carnelian is thought to support the digestive system by improving metabolism and promoting healthy digestion. It is often used for conditions like bloating, constipation, or low appetite, helping to restore balance to the digestive tract.

6. Selenite for Detoxification and Pain Relief

Selenite is known for its purifying and detoxifying qualities, making it beneficial for those seeking relief from inflammation or pain. It is often used to cleanse the body of negative energy and support the body's natural healing processes. Selenite is believed to help remove physical blockages in the energy field, which can contribute to chronic pain or discomfort. It is also used for conditions like arthritis, muscle soreness, or joint pain, as it is thought to promote cellular regeneration and reduce inflammation. Placing selenite over affected areas can help ease pain and support healing.

7. Lapis Lazuli for Mental Clarity and Pain Relief

Lapis lazuli is primarily known for its ability to enhance mental clarity and communication, but it also has applications for physical healing. It is believed to be useful for relieving pain, particularly tension-related discomfort in the neck, shoulders, and head. Lapis lazuli works by releasing energetic blockages, promoting relaxation, and reducing emotional stress, which can contribute to physical tension and pain. It is also used to support the immune system and alleviate symptoms of colds or flu. When placed on sore or tight areas of the body, lapis lazuli is thought to aid in muscle relaxation and reduce discomfort.

8. Fluorite for Immune System and Skin Health

Fluorite is a powerful cleansing and detoxifying stone that can be beneficial for both the immune system and skin health. It is believed to purify the body by removing toxins and supporting the body's natural detoxification processes. Fluorite is thought to aid in the prevention of infections and support the body's ability to heal from illnesses. Additionally, it is said to promote healthy skin by addressing issues such as acne, eczema, or inflammation. Using fluorite in healing practices can help balance the body's energy, clear blockages, and encourage optimal health and vitality.

9. Black Tourmaline for Pain and Inflammation

Black tourmaline is a grounding stone known for its protective properties, but it also has therapeutic effects on physical health. It is commonly used to relieve pain and inflammation, particularly in the joints or muscles. Black tourmaline is thought to draw out negative energy and reduce stress, which can exacerbate chronic pain or inflammation. By grounding excess energy, black tourmaline helps to restore balance and promote healing in the body. It is also useful for alleviating symptoms of sciatica, arthritis, and other inflammatory conditions. Placing black tourmaline over affected areas or wearing it as jewelry can help reduce discomfort and enhance the body's natural healing processes.

10. Malachite for Joint and Muscle Pain

Malachite is a potent crystal often used for joint and muscle pain relief. It is believed to have anti-inflammatory properties that help soothe conditions like arthritis, back pain, or general muscle soreness. Malachite works by enhancing circulation and reducing swelling, which helps to alleviate discomfort in the affected areas. It is also thought to support the regeneration of tissues and promote the healing of injuries. Malachite can be placed directly on the body or worn as jewelry to offer continuous support for those suffering from chronic pain or inflammation.

11. Garnet for Blood Circulation and Vitality

Garnet is a deep red stone known for its ability to stimulate circulation and promote overall vitality. It is thought to increase energy levels, enhance physical strength, and improve the health of the circulatory system. Garnet is especially useful for those experiencing symptoms of anemia, poor circulation, or fatigue. By stimulating blood flow and oxygenation, garnet can help to improve energy levels, support physical endurance, and promote a general sense of well-being. Wearing garnet or carrying it with you can help boost your overall vitality and keep energy flowing freely through the body.

Conclusion

Crystals can be a valuable complement to traditional medical treatments, offering a natural way to address a variety of physical ailments. Whether used to relieve pain, reduce inflammation, support circulation, or aid in detoxification, each crystal has unique properties that may help promote physical healing and wellness. While crystals should not be relied upon as a sole treatment, incorporating them into your healing practices can provide additional support for the body's natural ability to recover and maintain optimal health. By choosing the right crystals for your specific physical needs, you can tap into their energetic properties to enhance your overall well-being.

Using Crystals for Detoxification

Crystals are believed to have powerful detoxifying properties that can support the body in clearing out toxins, both physical and energetic. Detoxification is a natural process that the body undergoes to eliminate harmful substances, but sometimes the system can become overwhelmed, especially in today's toxic environment. Crystal healing offers an alternative or complementary approach to assist with this process, helping to cleanse the body, mind, and spirit. By interacting with the body's energy fields, certain crystals are thought to promote the release of accumulated negative energies and support overall wellness.

1. Clear Quartz: Master Detoxifier

Clear quartz is often regarded as the most versatile crystal in detoxification practices. Known as the "master healer," clear quartz is believed to amplify energy and enhance the body's natural detoxifying abilities. Its purifying energy helps clear out negative energies, allowing for a fresh flow of positive vibrations. It can be used to detoxify both the body and the mind by promoting mental clarity and emotional balance. Placing clear quartz near the body or in your environment may help to stimulate the body's natural healing processes, supporting the elimination of toxins and promoting overall vitality.

2. Selenite: Energy Cleansing and Purification

Selenite is a highly effective crystal for detoxification, particularly for cleansing the energetic body. Its powerful purifying properties help to clear stagnant or negative energy, allowing for the release of blockages that could prevent the body from detoxifying effectively. Selenite is also known for its ability to cleanse other crystals, making it an essential tool in a detoxification practice. When used during meditation or placed on areas of the body that need healing, selenite is thought to support the removal of toxins on a physical level, encouraging purification and promoting cellular regeneration.

3. Black Tourmaline: Protective Detoxifier

Black tourmaline is primarily known for its protective and grounding properties, but it is also highly regarded for its detoxifying abilities. This stone is believed to absorb negative energies, environmental pollutants, and electromagnetic radiation (EMFs), which can contribute to a build-up of toxins in the body. By grounding excess energy and neutralizing harmful forces, black tourmaline helps to create a balanced, clean energy field around the body. This purification is thought to support the body's own detoxification systems, including the lymphatic and circulatory systems, helping to eliminate impurities and promote better health.

4. Amethyst: Calming Detox for the Mind and Body

Amethyst is not only a powerful crystal for mental clarity and emotional healing, but it is also a gentle detoxifier. It is believed to help clear out toxic emotions and mental patterns, providing support for emotional detoxification. On a physical level, amethyst is said to assist in the removal of toxins by stimulating the immune system and supporting liver function, which plays a crucial role in detoxification. Placing amethyst near the body or on the throat and third eye chakras can encourage a sense of calm while helping to purify both the mind and the physical body.

5. Fluorite: Cleanse and Detoxify

Fluorite is one of the most effective crystals for detoxification due to its ability to cleanse the body and mind of negative or stagnant energies. Fluorite is thought to help the body rid itself of toxins and pollutants by supporting the lymphatic system and the immune system. It is also believed to promote the detoxification of the digestive tract, helping with issues like bloating, constipation, and indigestion. Fluorite is also known for its ability to clear mental fog and bring focus, making it beneficial for those looking to clear out negative thought patterns while physically detoxifying.

6. Citrine: Cleansing for the Digestive System

Citrine is known for its bright, sunny energy and its ability to detoxify the body, particularly the digestive system. It is thought to stimulate the flow of energy in the solar plexus chakra, which is associated with digestion, metabolism, and personal power. Citrine can be used to support the body's detoxification process by aiding in the removal of waste and toxins through the digestive and urinary systems. It also helps to balance blood sugar levels, which can be beneficial during a detox process. Its energizing properties can help combat the fatigue often associated with detoxing, providing the stamina and motivation needed to stick with a cleanse.

7. Malachite: Deep Detox for the Physical Body

Malachite is a stone often used for deep detoxification, particularly for physical ailments like inflammation, joint pain, or digestive issues. It is believed to be highly effective in promoting the body's natural detox processes by supporting the liver, kidneys, and digestive system. Malachite is said to help clear toxins from the body and promote the flow of energy, which can lead to improved circulation and overall vitality. Its vibrant green color is associated with the heart chakra, and it is thought to enhance physical and emotional healing by releasing emotional blockages and encouraging deep cleansing.

8. Carnelian: Detox and Revitalization

Carnelian is a powerful stone for revitalizing and energizing the body. It stimulates the root and sacral chakras, which are associated with physical vitality, creativity, and action. In detox practices, carnelian is believed to support the body's natural metabolic functions, helping to stimulate digestion, improve circulation, and enhance the removal of toxins from the body. It is often used to invigorate the body during a cleanse or detox program, combating fatigue and boosting energy levels. Carnelian's revitalizing properties also promote emotional healing, helping to release stagnant or negative emotions that may be preventing the body from detoxifying properly.

9. Lapis Lazuli: Detoxification for the Mind and Body

Lapis lazuli, with its deep blue hue, is known for its ability to detoxify the mind and body. It is thought to help clear the mind of negative thought patterns, promoting mental clarity and focus. On a physical level, lapis lazuli is believed to support the detoxification of the liver and other organs involved in cleansing the body. It is also thought to help with respiratory issues, supporting the body in clearing out toxins from the lungs. Lapis lazuli is often used to relieve stress and anxiety, which can contribute to emotional blockages that hinder the body's ability to detoxify effectively.

10. Smoky Quartz: Grounding Detoxification

Smoky quartz is a grounding stone known for its ability to absorb and neutralize negative energies, including physical toxins and emotional blockages. It is believed to support the body's detoxification processes by helping to release impurities from the body and mind. Smoky quartz is thought to clear stagnant energies, making space for healing and renewal. It is also said to protect against environmental pollutants and electromagnetic radiation, both of which can contribute to toxic build-up in the body. By wearing smoky quartz or keeping it nearby during detoxification, you can enhance the process of cleansing and purification on all levels.

11. Rose Quartz: Gentle Detox for Emotional Healing

While rose quartz is primarily associated with emotional healing, it also supports detoxification by encouraging the release of toxic emotional energy. It is often used to heal the heart chakra, helping to release past traumas, grief, and negative emotional patterns. Rose quartz's calming energy assists in emotional detoxification, allowing for the gentle removal of toxic feelings such as anger, jealousy, or sadness. By addressing the emotional aspects of detoxification, rose quartz can help to create a more balanced and harmonious state of being, which in turn supports the physical detox process.

Conclusion

Using crystals for detoxification can be a powerful way to support the body's natural cleansing and healing processes. Each crystal offers unique properties that can aid in the removal of physical toxins, negative energies, and emotional blockages, allowing for a deeper, more holistic detox. Whether you are looking to cleanse your body, mind, or spirit, crystals like clear quartz, selenite, fluorite, and amethyst can provide valuable support in your detox journey. By incorporating these stones into your routine—whether through meditation, wearing them as jewelry, or placing them on specific areas of the body—you can enhance your detoxification process and foster greater overall health and well-being.

Crystal Healing for Mental Clarity

Mental clarity is an essential aspect of overall well-being, and many individuals seek ways to clear mental fog, enhance focus, and improve decision-making. Crystal healing offers a natural and non-invasive approach to support mental clarity by interacting with the energy field and stimulating the brain's natural processes. Certain crystals are believed to possess unique properties that can help clear blockages, balance emotions, and enhance cognitive function, allowing the mind to operate at its fullest potential.

1. Clear Quartz: Amplifier of Mental Focus

Clear quartz is one of the most powerful crystals for promoting mental clarity. Known as the "master healer," clear quartz is believed to amplify energy and focus the mind. It helps to clear negative or stagnant energy, which can cloud judgment and interfere with concentration. By amplifying positive energy, clear quartz can help individuals stay focused, organized, and clear-headed, especially in situations that require decision-making or critical thinking. Whether placed on the third eye or crown chakra, clear quartz is used to stimulate mental faculties and enhance concentration, making it a favorite among those looking to boost cognitive function.

2. Amethyst: Calming and Clarity-Enhancing

Amethyst is known for its calming properties, which are essential for achieving mental clarity. This crystal helps quiet the mind and soothe anxiety, allowing for better concentration and focus. Amethyst is often used to enhance meditation, making it easier to enter a state of calmness and clear thought. It is also said to assist in breaking through mental blockages that can cause confusion or mental fatigue. The crystal's soothing energy helps create a serene environment, ideal for clarity of thought, and fosters a sense of peace that promotes better decision-making.

3. Fluorite: Mental Detox and Focus

Fluorite is a powerful crystal for clearing mental fog and promoting mental clarity. Known for its ability to cleanse and detoxify, fluorite is believed to help remove negative energies and confusion that may be clouding the mind. It is particularly useful when someone is feeling overwhelmed, scattered, or unable to focus. Fluorite's energy is thought to improve concentration and mental organization, making it ideal for those studying, working on projects, or tackling complex tasks. This crystal's ability to clear mental blockages also aids in opening up new pathways for creative and rational thinking.

4. Lapis Lazuli: Enhancing Wisdom and Insight

Lapis lazuli is traditionally known as a stone of wisdom and truth. It is thought to promote mental clarity by stimulating the mind, increasing intellectual abilities, and enhancing intuition. This crystal supports mental acuity and the ability to understand complex ideas, making it ideal for individuals looking to enhance their problem-solving skills or gain insight into challenging situations. Lapis lazuli is also believed to foster a deeper connection with one's inner self, allowing for greater self-awareness and clarity in decision-making. Its strong energetic connection to the third eye and throat chakras makes it particularly effective for improving communication and mental expression.

5. Citrine: Energizing the Mind

Citrine is often associated with abundance and success, but it also has powerful effects on mental clarity. Known for its energizing properties, citrine is believed to uplift the mind and stimulate positive mental energy. It helps to clear mental clutter and promote clear thinking, making it useful for individuals who need to remain sharp and focused throughout the day. Citrine's cheerful, sunny energy encourages optimism, which can be helpful in maintaining a positive mindset and overcoming feelings of doubt or confusion. By aligning the solar plexus chakra, citrine also supports personal empowerment, enabling individuals to make decisions with confidence and clarity.

6. Sodalite: Rational Thinking and Calmness

Sodalite is a crystal that helps to balance the logical and intuitive mind, making it ideal for promoting mental clarity. It is often used to facilitate rational thinking and communication, providing the clarity needed to make clear, informed decisions. Sodalite is thought to enhance one's ability to think critically, organize thoughts, and solve problems. It also promotes a calm, peaceful state of mind, helping to reduce mental stress and anxiety that can cloud judgment. By balancing the throat and third eye chakras, sodalite supports clear expression and a more grounded approach to decision-making.

7. Tiger's Eye: Grounding and Mental Clarity

Tiger's eye is a grounding crystal that is often used to bring clarity and focus during stressful situations. It is particularly helpful for overcoming mental blockages and doubts, allowing for a more balanced and clear-thinking approach to challenges. Tiger's eye helps stimulate both the root and solar plexus chakras, promoting a sense of stability and confidence. It encourages practical thinking, enhancing decision-making and problem-solving abilities. This crystal is also said to promote a clear mind by dispelling distractions and helping to sharpen focus during complex or multitasking activities.

8. Black Tourmaline: Clearing Mental Blockages

Black tourmaline is primarily known for its protective properties, but it also has benefits for mental clarity. This crystal is believed to help clear mental blockages and protect against negative energies that can disrupt clear thinking. Black tourmaline supports the grounding of the mind, encouraging focus and mental organization. It is often used to eliminate distractions, reduce anxiety, and promote a state of calm clarity. Its grounding nature helps to stabilize emotional turbulence, allowing the mind to function clearly and efficiently.

9. Rose Quartz: Emotional Clarity and Calm

While rose quartz is best known for its emotional healing properties, it also helps to foster mental clarity by addressing emotional blockages. Emotional baggage, such as unresolved grief or stress, can cloud one's judgment and interfere with clear thinking. Rose quartz helps to open the heart chakra, promoting emotional balance and self-compassion. When emotions are balanced, mental clarity improves, and decision-making becomes easier. Rose quartz fosters a peaceful, loving state of mind, which supports mental clarity and positive thinking in both personal and professional matters.

10. Aquamarine: Calm and Clear Communication

Aquamarine is a soothing crystal that helps to enhance both mental clarity and communication skills. It is often used to calm the mind and reduce stress, which can contribute to mental fog and confusion. Aquamarine's gentle energy helps individuals approach difficult situations with a calm and open mind, promoting clarity in communication. This crystal also supports mental relaxation, making it useful for individuals looking to unwind and clear their minds before engaging in important conversations or making decisions. Aquamarine is particularly effective for those in leadership roles or positions where clear, thoughtful communication is essential.

11. Amazonite: Enhancing Clarity Through Communication

Amazonite is often used to promote clear, truthful communication and to remove emotional blockages that may hinder mental clarity. By calming the nervous system and reducing anxiety, amazonite creates space for clearer thoughts and better decision-making. It supports the throat chakra, helping individuals express themselves more clearly, and encourages open-mindedness. This crystal is ideal for those who need mental clarity to communicate ideas effectively or who are facing challenging conversations. It is also thought to foster a balanced state of mind, reducing confusion and mental stress.

Conclusion

Crystals can be valuable tools for enhancing mental clarity, helping to clear away distractions, emotional blockages, and negative energy that may cloud judgment or hinder focus. Each crystal carries its unique energy that interacts with the body's energy system to support cognitive function and clarity. Whether you are looking to improve concentration, reduce mental fog, or foster better decision-making, crystals like clear quartz, amethyst, fluorite, and lapis lazuli offer powerful support. By incorporating crystals into your daily routine—whether through meditation, carrying them as pocket stones, or placing them around your workspace—you can create an environment that promotes mental focus, clear thinking, and improved cognitive performance.

Crystals for Concentration and Memory

Concentration and memory are vital components of cognitive function, impacting everything from learning and problem-solving to daily tasks and decision-making. In the realm of crystal healing, certain stones are believed to enhance mental clarity, improve focus, and boost memory retention. By interacting with the body's energy system, these crystals are thought to support brain function, stimulate the mind, and promote mental sharpness. Whether you are studying for exams, working on a project, or simply seeking to improve your cognitive performance, crystals can offer valuable assistance in strengthening concentration and memory.

1. Fluorite: Clarity and Mental Organization

Fluorite is known for its ability to clear mental fog and improve mental organization. It is believed to stimulate the brain and enhance concentration, helping to clear distractions and improve focus. Fluorite is often used to improve memory retention by clearing away stagnant energies that may cloud the mind. It helps the mind stay clear and organized, making it easier to process and retain information. Fluorite's energetic properties support mental clarity and boost the ability to recall important details, making it an excellent choice for anyone looking to sharpen their memory.

2. Clear Quartz: Amplifier of Focus

Clear quartz is one of the most versatile crystals in the healing world. Known as a "master healer," it amplifies energy and enhances mental clarity, making it a popular choice for improving concentration and memory. By clearing mental fog and focusing the mind, clear quartz is thought to increase cognitive abilities and improve overall mental performance. Whether used during meditation, placed on the crown chakra, or carried as a pocket stone, clear quartz supports focused thinking and helps the brain retain and process information more efficiently.

3. Lapis Lazuli: Stimulating the Mind

Lapis lazuli is a powerful stone for enhancing intellectual abilities and memory. It stimulates the third eye and throat chakras, which are associated with higher mental faculties and clear communication. Lapis lazuli is thought to support critical thinking, problem-solving, and memory recall, making it an excellent choice for anyone involved in learning or creative work. Its energetic properties help to enhance concentration and reduce mental clutter, allowing the mind to focus more effectively. Lapis lazuli is also believed to encourage insight and wisdom, helping individuals access deeper knowledge stored within their subconscious.

4. Carnelian: Boosting Motivation and Focus

Carnelian is a vibrant, energizing stone that stimulates both the root and sacral chakras. It is known for its ability to boost motivation, drive, and focus. Carnelian enhances concentration by helping the mind stay alert and energized, making it easier to stay engaged in tasks for extended periods. It also helps increase the flow of energy to the brain, stimulating memory retention and cognitive function. For those who struggle with procrastination or mental fatigue, carnelian's invigorating energy can provide the boost needed to stay focused and on track.

5. Amethyst: Enhancing Mental Clarity

Amethyst is often used to calm the mind and relieve stress, which can hinder concentration and memory. By soothing anxiety and promoting a peaceful mental state, amethyst helps improve the ability to focus and remember important details. It is also believed to stimulate the third eye chakra, enhancing intuition and mental clarity. This makes amethyst a great choice for improving both concentration and memory. It helps create a calm and balanced mental environment, allowing for clearer thinking and better retention of information.

6. Sodalite: Rational Thinking and Focused Mind

Sodalite is known for its ability to enhance rational thinking and improve concentration. This crystal stimulates the throat and third eye chakras, supporting clear thought, communication, and mental focus. Sodalite helps reduce mental confusion, promoting a clear and organized state of mind. It is particularly useful for those studying, working on intellectual tasks, or trying to improve memory recall. By boosting mental organization and clarity, sodalite aids in both remembering information and staying mentally alert during demanding tasks.

7. Tiger's Eye: Enhancing Focus and Practicality

Tiger's eye is a grounding and stabilizing stone that supports mental clarity and concentration. It enhances focus by reducing distractions and helping the mind stay centered. Tiger's eye is often used to increase practical thinking, making it easier to apply learned information to real-world situations. It also supports memory retention by improving mental organization and helping individuals recall information when needed.

For those who need to stay focused on long-term goals, tiger's eye provides the discipline and mental strength to stay on track.

8. Citrine: Uplifting the Mind

Citrine is a bright, uplifting stone that enhances energy and focus. Its stimulating energy helps combat mental fatigue, making it easier to concentrate on tasks for longer periods. Citrine is also believed to improve memory retention by enhancing mental clarity and focus. As a stone of abundance and personal empowerment, citrine encourages a positive mindset, helping individuals stay motivated and alert. By stimulating the solar plexus chakra, citrine boosts mental energy and concentration, which can lead to improved memory and cognitive function.

9. Rose Quartz: Healing the Mind for Clarity

While rose quartz is primarily known for its emotional healing properties, it can also help improve concentration and memory by addressing emotional blockages that may be affecting mental clarity. Stress, anxiety, and emotional turmoil can cloud the mind and make it harder to focus or retain information. Rose quartz helps to release emotional tension and promote a peaceful state of mind, allowing the brain to function more effectively. It also promotes self-compassion and emotional balance, reducing mental distractions and improving overall concentration.

10. Amazonite: Clear Communication and Focus

Amazonite is a soothing stone that promotes clear communication and mental clarity. It is believed to reduce stress and anxiety, which can hinder the ability to focus and remember information. Amazonite helps calm the mind, allowing for better concentration and improved mental performance. By balancing the throat chakra, it enhances verbal expression and helps individuals articulate their thoughts more clearly. This can be particularly helpful when studying, engaging in intellectual discussions, or working on tasks that require mental sharpness.

11. Malachite: Deep Thinking and Focus

Malachite is known for its ability to stimulate deep thinking and focus. It is thought to help clear the mind of negative thought patterns and mental clutter, enabling better concentration. Malachite enhances memory recall by clearing emotional blockages and allowing the mind to function at its highest potential. This crystal is also believed to help individuals access and retain important information more easily, making it ideal for learning and intellectual pursuits.

Conclusion

Crystals can be a powerful tool for improving concentration and memory. Whether you are looking to enhance focus during work, study for exams, or simply improve mental performance, certain stones like fluorite, clear quartz, lapis lazuli, and carnelian can support your cognitive function. By stimulating the brain, clearing mental fog, and reducing emotional distractions, these crystals help create an environment conducive to better concentration and memory retention. Incorporating crystals into your daily routine—whether through meditation, wearing them as jewelry, or placing them in your workspace—can offer lasting support for boosting mental clarity and cognitive abilities.

Crystals for Creativity and Inspiration

Creativity and inspiration are vital forces in artistic endeavors, problem-solving, and personal growth. Crystals, with their unique energetic properties, are often used to enhance these qualities, helping individuals unlock their creative potential, spark new ideas, and find the motivation needed to bring those ideas to life. Whether you're an artist, writer, entrepreneur, or anyone seeking to tap into your creative flow, certain crystals are believed to offer valuable support by stimulating the mind, clearing blockages, and encouraging innovative thinking.

1. Citrine: Energizing Creativity

Citrine is a bright, energizing crystal that stimulates creativity and imagination. Known for its cheerful, uplifting energy, citrine encourages a positive mindset, making it easier to access creative ideas. This crystal is believed to clear mental blockages, boost self-confidence, and promote a sense of abundance, which is essential for creative expression. Citrine also works to open the solar plexus chakra, the center of personal power, which enhances motivation and encourages individuals to take action on their creative ideas. It is particularly useful when seeking to overcome self-doubt and jump-start new projects.

2. Carnelian: Boosting Artistic Expression

Carnelian is often referred to as a stone of action and creativity. Known for its warm, fiery energy, it stimulates both the root and sacral chakras, which are linked to passion, creativity, and sensuality. Carnelian is believed to ignite motivation and inspire new ideas, making it ideal for artists, musicians, writers, and anyone engaged in creative pursuits. It helps combat procrastination by boosting confidence and providing the energy needed to bring creative ideas into action. Carnelian also enhances the ability to express oneself, making it a valuable tool for artists seeking to communicate their visions and emotions through their work.

3. Amethyst: Unlocking Intuition and Inspiration

Amethyst is known for its connection to higher states of consciousness, making it an excellent crystal for enhancing creativity and spiritual inspiration. This stone is believed to stimulate the third eye and crown chakras, which are associated with intuition, imagination, and connection to higher wisdom. Amethyst encourages individuals to tap into their inner creative potential by facilitating a deeper connection with their subconscious mind. It is particularly beneficial for those seeking to enhance their intuitive creativity or to break through mental blocks that stifle artistic expression. Amethyst can help bring clarity to creative ideas and encourage innovative thinking.

4. Lapis Lazuli: Expanding Imagination

Lapis lazuli is a stone of wisdom and truth, known for its ability to stimulate creativity by unlocking the imagination. This crystal activates the third eye and throat chakras, promoting clear communication, self-expression, and deep thinking. Lapis lazuli is particularly effective for those working on projects that require original thinking or innovative problem-solving. It is often used by writers, artists, and musicians to enhance their ability to think outside the box and push creative boundaries. By fostering a sense of clarity and inner vision, lapis lazuli helps individuals access deeper layers of creativity and inspiration.

5. Fluorite: Mental Clarity for Creative Flow

Fluorite is a powerful crystal for clearing mental fog and enhancing concentration, making it an excellent stone for promoting creativity. It is believed to help clear the mind of distractions and mental clutter, allowing for greater mental focus and the ability to bring creative ideas into fruition. Fluorite's energy supports mental organization, helping individuals make sense of complex ideas and bring structure to creative projects. By clearing energetic blockages, fluorite helps the creative flow move more freely, enabling new ideas to emerge with clarity and precision.

6. Rose Quartz: Opening the Heart to Creative Expression

Rose quartz is often associated with love and compassion, but it also plays a crucial role in unlocking creativity. This gentle crystal helps to open the heart chakra, promoting emotional healing and self-love. When the heart is open and free of emotional blockages, individuals can express themselves more authentically, which is key to creative expression. Rose quartz encourages a nurturing environment that supports creativity, helping individuals connect with their emotions and express them through art, writing, or other creative endeavors. It also helps to foster a sense of inner peace, which can enhance inspiration and motivation.

7. Tiger's Eye: Balancing Creativity and Practicality

Tiger's eye is a grounding stone known for its ability to balance creativity with practicality. It stimulates the sacral chakra, which governs creativity, and the solar plexus chakra, which influences personal power and action. Tiger's eye provides the focus and determination needed to see creative projects through to completion, making it a great stone for those who struggle with turning creative ideas into tangible outcomes. By enhancing both creative thinking and practical action, tiger's eye ensures that inspiration is not only sparked but also brought to fruition with clear intent.

8. Amazonite: Encouraging Honest Expression

Amazonite is a crystal that promotes creativity through clear, honest communication and expression. It activates both the throat and heart chakras, allowing individuals to express their feelings and ideas freely without fear of judgment. This makes it an excellent crystal for creative work that requires vulnerability and authenticity. Whether you're an artist, writer, or performer, amazonite encourages you to speak from the heart and create without inhibition It helps reduce anxiety and self-doubt, making it easier to access the creative flow and share your unique perspective with the world.

9. Green Aventurine: Inspiring New Ideas

Green aventurine is a stone of opportunity, known for its ability to stimulate growth and bring new ideas to the forefront. Often referred to as the "stone of luck," green aventurine is believed to enhance creativity by creating a positive, abundant environment for new ideas to flourish. This crystal encourages a mindset of possibility and potential, making it easier to access inspiration and take creative risks. Green aventurine is also a great stone for those embarking on new creative ventures, as it helps promote optimism and a positive outlook on the future

10. Smoky Quartz: Grounding Creative Energy

Smoky quartz is a grounding crystal that helps anchor creative energy, ensuring that ideas are rooted in practicality and manifest in the material world. This crystal is especially beneficial for those who may feel overwhelmed by the influx of ideas or creativity and need help grounding those thoughts into actionable plans. Smoky quartz's calming energy helps dispel negativity, reduce anxiety, and keep the mind clear, allowing for a balanced flow of creative energy. By stabilizing and protecting the creative process, smoky quartz ensures that inspiration can be nurtured and brought to fruition.

11. Peacock Ore: Enhancing Artistic Vision

Peacock ore, also known as bornite, is a vibrant crystal known for its ability to enhance artistic vision and inspire creativity. Its shimmering, iridescent colors are thought to stimulate the third eye chakra, encouraging vivid imagination and inspiration. Peacock ore is believed to help break through creative blocks and encourage new ways of thinking. It is especially useful for those who feel "stuck" in their creative pursuits and need a spark to ignite their artistic flow. This crystal's vibrant energy fosters a deeper connection with the creative self and inspires new ideas.

Conclusion

Crystals offer a powerful way to enhance creativity and inspire new ideas by aligning with the body's energy fields and encouraging a harmonious flow of inspiration. Whether you're an artist looking to push your boundaries, a writer searching for fresh ideas, or anyone seeking to unlock their full creative potential, crystals like citrine, carnelian, lapis lazuli, and fluorite can provide the support and energy needed to ignite the creative process. By using these crystals, individuals can clear blockages, enhance mental clarity, and connect more deeply with their inner creative power, leading to innovative, inspired work.

Crystals for Stress and Anxiety

Stress and anxiety are common experiences that affect both the mind and body. They can manifest in various forms, from general feelings of unease to intense panic attacks, and they often interfere with daily life. Crystal healing has been used as a natural remedy to help alleviate stress and anxiety by balancing the body's energy, calming the nervous system, and promoting emotional well-being. Many crystals are thought to have soothing, grounding, or energizing properties that can help reduce the intensity of stress and restore inner calm. Here are some crystals commonly used to address stress and anxiety:

1. Amethyst: Calm and Clarity

Amethyst is one of the most popular crystals for reducing stress and anxiety. Known for its calming energy, amethyst is said to soothe the mind and relieve emotional tension. It is believed to help reduce anxiety by quieting the overactive thoughts that often accompany stress. Amethyst also promotes a sense of peace, making it a valuable tool for individuals who suffer from insomnia or restless thoughts. By stimulating the crown and third eye chakras, amethyst helps increase spiritual awareness, enabling a sense of clarity and calm. It can be particularly effective in managing stress caused by emotional or spiritual turmoil.

2. Rose Quartz: Emotional Healing and Peace

Rose quartz is widely known for its ability to open and heal the heart chakra, promoting love, compassion, and emotional balance. It is particularly useful for managing stress and anxiety related to relationships, self-esteem, and unresolved emotional wounds. Rose quartz is believed to help release negative emotions, replace fear with love, and encourage self-care. Its gentle energy soothes the heart and calms the mind, allowing individuals to navigate stressful situations with more compassion and understanding. Rose quartz is also known to help reduce the emotional tension that often accompanies anxiety.

3. Lepidolite: The Stress-Reliever

Lepidolite is known for its powerful ability to alleviate stress and anxiety. It contains high amounts of lithium, which is a key component of many antidepressants. Lepidolite's calming and soothing energy is particularly effective in managing feelings of overwhelm and emotional instability. It is often used to ease feelings of panic, sadness, and emotional imbalance. Lepidolite is said to calm the nervous system, helping individuals feel grounded and centered in the midst of stressful or anxiety-inducing situations. It's a go-to crystal for emotional healing and mental clarity, making it ideal for times of heightened stress.

4. Black Tourmaline: Grounding and Protection

Black tourmaline is a powerful protective stone that helps ground and stabilize the body's energy. It is particularly effective for those who experience anxiety caused by external factors, such as overwhelming environments or negative energies. Black tourmaline is believed to absorb and deflect negative energy, creating a shield of protection around the individual. This grounding stone helps alleviate feelings of fear and insecurity, promoting a sense of stability and calm. It is also useful for helping to reduce stress caused by overthinking or feeling disconnected from reality.

5. Sodalite: Mental Clarity and Calm

Sodalite is known for its ability to promote mental clarity and calm the mind. By stimulating the throat and third eye chakras, sodalite supports effective communication and rational thinking. It is especially useful for people who experience anxiety due to mental overwhelm or excessive worry. Sodalite helps release negative thought patterns, promoting a sense of inner peace and balance. It also encourages emotional balance by helping individuals process their emotions logically and with a calm perspective, reducing emotional turbulence and mental stress.

6. Howlite: Reducing Anxiety and Overthinking

Howlite is a soothing stone that helps reduce anxiety, stress, and overthinking. It is known for its calming energy, which helps quiet the mind and promote relaxation. Howlite is particularly helpful for individuals who suffer from insomnia or restless thoughts, as it aids in promoting restful sleep and emotional peace. Its calming influence helps prevent the mind from spiraling into anxiety and fear, making it an excellent stone for those who need help managing overwhelming emotions. Howlite also encourages patience and understanding, which can be particularly beneficial for navigating stressful or challenging situations.

7. Aventurine: Calming and Soothing Energy

Green aventurine is a crystal that promotes emotional healing and brings a sense of calm and stability. Known as the "Stone of Opportunity," aventurine is believed to help release feelings of frustration and anxiety, especially when they are related to external pressures or perceived setbacks. Its gentle energy helps to soothe the nervous system, reduce stress, and encourage a sense of emotional balance. Aventurine is also said to help ease feelings of heartache or grief, making it a good choice for emotional healing in times of distress.

8. Clear Quartz: Amplifier of Calm

Clear quartz is a versatile crystal that can be used in combination with other stones to amplify their calming properties. It is known for its ability to cleanse the energy around it, remove blockages, and promote balance. Clear quartz is said to work in harmony with other crystals, enhancing their energy and helping to stabilize the emotional body. It can also promote clarity and focus, helping individuals break free from anxious thoughts and regain mental control. Clear quartz encourages overall healing, making it an excellent tool for stress reduction and emotional well-being.

9. Moonstone: Emotional Harmony and Stress Relief

Moonstone is a crystal that helps balance emotions and promotes inner peace. Known for its soothing and calming properties, moonstone is said to relieve stress by encouraging emotional balance. It is particularly effective in addressing anxiety that stems from hormonal imbalances or mood swings. Moonstone works with the sacral chakra, helping to release emotional tension and allowing individuals to process feelings without being overwhelmed by them. Its gentle energy also promotes rest and relaxation, making it an ideal stone for easing stress before bedtime.

10. Chrysoprase: Comfort and Calm

Chrysoprase is a stone of emotional healing that is often used to alleviate feelings of anxiety and stress. Its calming energy is said to help clear emotional blockages and promote feelings of well-being. Chrysoprase encourages a sense of emotional security and helps ease fear, tension, and anxiety. It also supports emotional recovery and healing, making it particularly beneficial for those dealing with emotional trauma or feelings of abandonment. Chrysoprase's soothing properties help individuals feel safe and supported, allowing them to navigate stress with a calm, peaceful mindset.

Conclusion

Crystals have been used for centuries to alleviate stress and anxiety by working with the body's energy system. Stones such as amethyst, rose quartz, lepidolite, and black tourmaline are believed to help calm the mind, soothe emotional turmoil, and promote a sense of peace and grounding. Whether you're looking for a stone to reduce anxiety in stressful situations or to help release emotional tension over time, these crystals can offer significant support. By integrating these stones into your daily life—whether through meditation, carrying them with you, or placing them in your environment—you can create a calming, supportive energy that helps reduce the impact of stress and anxiety on your well-being.

How to Program Your Crystals with Intention

Crystals are powerful tools in healing and energy work, but their full potential is often unlocked when they are programmed with a specific intention. Programming a crystal involves infusing it with a purpose or goal, allowing it to align with your personal energy and support your desires, whether for healing, manifestation, or spiritual growth. The process is simple and intuitive, yet profoundly impactful, as it taps into the crystal's unique energetic properties and channels them toward your specific needs.

1. Choose Your Crystal

The first step in programming a crystal is selecting the right one for your intention. Each crystal has its own unique energy, and some are better suited for specific purposes. For example, amethyst is often chosen for spiritual growth and calm, while rose quartz is used for love and emotional healing. Citrine is commonly used for abundance and manifestation, and black tourmaline is a powerful protector against negative energies. Choose a crystal that resonates with your goal and intuition, as this will enhance the effectiveness of the programming.

2. Cleanse Your Crystal

Before programming a crystal, it's important to cleanse it to remove any lingering energies it may have absorbed from previous uses. Crystals can absorb both positive and negative energy, so cleaning them ensures that they are energetically clear and ready to be programmed with your intention. There are various methods for cleansing crystals, including:

- **Smudging** with sage, palo santo, or incense to purify the crystal's energy.
- **Running water**, especially under a stream of natural water like a river or creek (ensure the crystal is safe to be exposed to water).
- **Placing the crystal under the moonlight**, particularly during a full moon, which is believed to cleanse and recharge the stone.
- **Using sound**, such as a tuning fork or singing bowl, to release negative energies from the crystal.

Once the crystal has been cleansed, it is ready to receive your intention.

3. Set Your Intention

The next step in programming your crystal is to set a clear, focused intention. This is where you align your desire or goal with the crystal's energy. Your intention should be specific, positive, and present tense. Instead of vague goals like "I want more money," try something more specific and actionable like, "I attract financial abundance with ease and grace." The clearer and more positive your intention, the more effective the programming will be.

To set your intention, hold the crystal in your hands and take a few deep breaths to center yourself. Clear your mind of any distractions and focus on what you want to achieve. Visualize your desired outcome and feel the emotions associated with it—whether it's peace, abundance, or health. Imagine your intention flowing into the crystal as you breathe deeply and connect with its energy.

4. Infuse the Crystal with Your Energy

Once you've set your intention, it's time to infuse the crystal with that energy. You can do this by holding the crystal in your hands, placing it over your heart or in your lap, and focusing your energy on it. As you focus, visualize your intention being absorbed by the crystal, enveloping it in the energy of your goal.

Some people like to speak their intention aloud while holding the crystal, affirming their desires with words like, "I program this crystal to help me manifest love and compassion" or "This crystal will bring me clarity and peace in difficult situations." Speaking your intention out loud can amplify its power and solidify your commitment to it.

You can also use visualization to further strengthen the programming. Imagine a bright light or energy flowing from your heart or mind and merging with the crystal, imbuing it with your desires. Some practitioners prefer to hold the crystal in their dominant hand (the hand they use to give energy) to channel energy directly into the stone, while others use both hands to create balance.

5. Trust and Let Go

After programming your crystal, it's important to trust that the energy is now aligned with your intention. Once you've infused the crystal with your goal, it's time to let go of any attachment to the outcome. Trust that the crystal will work on your behalf, and avoid obsessing over when or how your intention will manifest. The process of programming is as much about releasing control as it is about setting the energy in motion.

Place the crystal in a location where it will constantly remind you of your intention. This could be a personal space, your bedroom, your desk, or anywhere you can see it often. If you feel a connection with the crystal, you may also carry it with you, allowing its energy to accompany you throughout the day.

6. Reprogramming Your Crystal

Crystals can be reprogrammed whenever you feel the need to shift your focus or intention. If your desires change or if the crystal has been used for a different purpose, cleanse it and then set a new intention. You can program your crystal as often as you wish, making it a versatile tool that evolves with your needs.

7. How to Know if the Crystal is Working

You may begin to notice subtle signs that the crystal is working, such as changes in your emotions, thoughts, or circumstances. The process can be gradual, so patience is key. Pay attention to any synchronicities, feelings of peace, or new opportunities that arise, as these are often indicators that the crystal's energy is aligning with your intention.

Conclusion

Programming a crystal with intention is a powerful way to harness the unique energies of the stone and direct them toward your goals. Whether you are looking to heal, manifest abundance, find peace, or foster self-love, programming your crystal can enhance your connection to the energy you desire. The key is to approach the process with clarity, trust, and an open heart, allowing the crystal's vibrations to support your journey. By setting your intentions and aligning your energy with the crystal's, you create a harmonious relationship that helps manifest your desired outcome.

Techniques for Charging Your Crystals

Charging your crystals is an essential practice that ensures they remain energetically vibrant and effective. Crystals can absorb energy from their environment, and over time, they may become depleted or saturated, which can reduce their healing properties. Charging them helps restore their natural vibrancy, allowing them to work at their full potential. There are several methods for charging crystals, each aligning with different energies and intentions. Here are some of the most popular and effective techniques:

1. Moonlight

One of the most natural and widely used methods for charging crystals is to place them under the moonlight, particularly during a full moon. The full moon's energy is known for its cleansing and recharging properties, making it an ideal time to renew your crystals. Simply place your crystals outside or near a window where they can absorb the moon's light. This method is especially effective for calming stones like amethyst, selenite, and rose quartz, which benefit from the moon's soothing, gentle energy. For more powerful stones, like clear quartz, the full moon's energy helps amplify their properties. If the full moon is not visible, placing your crystals under a waxing or waning moon can still charge them with its subtle energy

2. Sunlight

Sunlight is another potent source for charging your crystals, providing a vibrant and energizing boost. Sunlight is ideal for stones that need revitalization, such as citrine, carnelian, and tiger's eye. The sun's rays are considered an excellent source of vitality and strength, and they work well for crystals associated with action, willpower, and manifestation. However, some crystals, particularly delicate stones like amethyst, rose quartz, and fluorite, may fade or become damaged when exposed to prolonged sunlight, so it's important to use caution when choosing this method. A few hours in the sun is often enough to recharge most crystals.

3. Earth Burial

Burying your crystals in the earth is one of the oldest and most traditional methods for charging them. The earth is a natural conductor of energy, and it can help ground and restore crystals by reconnecting them to the earth's energy field. To charge your crystals in the earth, find a safe outdoor spot (such as a garden or yard) and bury them a few inches below the surface. Leave them buried for a day or two, allowing the earth to cleanse and recharge the stone. This method is particularly effective for grounding stones like hematite, black tourmaline, and obsidian. When you retrieve the crystal, it will feel revitalized and reconnected to nature's grounding forces.

4. Selenite Charging Plate

Selenite is known for its cleansing and charging abilities, and it is often used to purify and recharge other crystals. A selenite charging plate or wand can be placed under or beside your crystals to restore their energy. Simply place your stones on the selenite surface for several hours or overnight. The selenite acts as a purifier, neutralizing any negative or stagnant energy and re-energizing your crystals. This is an ideal method for delicate stones that may not tolerate direct sunlight or water, such as lapis lazuli or moldavite. Selenite's energy works in a gentle, continuous flow, making it a safe and effective charging tool.

5. Sound and Vibrational Charging

Sound is a powerful method of clearing and charging crystals, as it works with vibrations to reset their energetic frequency. Tibetan singing bowls, tuning forks, or crystal sound bowls can all be used to create vibrational waves that help charge your stones. Each crystal has its own frequency, and sound can help realign it to its optimal energetic state. You can place your crystal near the source of the sound, such as in front of a singing bowl or tuning fork, or gently tap the bowl to let the sound fill the room. The sound waves create an energetic field that penetrates the crystal, restoring its energetic flow. This method is particularly effective for high-vibration stones like clear quartz and amethyst.

6. Water (For Certain Crystals)

Water is often used to cleanse crystals, but it can also be a useful tool for charging—provided the stone is water-safe. Stones like clear quartz, amethyst, citrine, and aquamarine can benefit from being submerged in clean water for a short period to revitalize their energy. To charge crystals in water, fill a bowl with spring water or natural water and submerge the crystals for several hours. The flowing energy of the water works to cleanse and charge the stone simultaneously. Be cautious, as some crystals, like selenite and malachite, are water-soluble and should not be exposed to moisture.

7. Crystal Clusters

Using a crystal cluster, especially one with a high energy frequency like quartz, is an effective way to charge individual stones. Place the crystal you wish to charge in the center of a cluster, allowing the cluster's energy to radiate outward and transfer to the stone. Crystal clusters, especially quartz and amethyst clusters, are self-charging and provide a continuous flow of energy. This method works well for maintaining the energy of crystals used for long-term healing or daily use. Crystal grids can also be created by arranging multiple stones in specific patterns to amplify their energy and recharge your crystals.

8. Visualization

Visualization is a powerful method of charging crystals using your mind's energy. Begin by holding the crystal in your hands and focusing on your breath. Close your eyes and imagine a bright light or energy flowing from your hands into the crystal, filling it with your intention. This method can be particularly useful for charging crystals when other options are not available, such as during travel. Visualization works by aligning the crystal's energy with your own, helping you to restore its frequency and purpose. For best results, use visualization in combination with other charging methods, like sunlight or sound.

9. Reiki and Energy Healing

Reiki practitioners or those skilled in energy healing can use their hands to direct energy into crystals. Reiki works by channeling universal life force energy to cleanse and recharge crystals. Hold the crystal in your hands or place it on a surface, and use your hands or focused intention to direct energy into the stone. The crystal will absorb this energy, which will help clear blockages and restore its natural vibrational state. Reiki charging can be done with a crystal grid, or each stone can be charged individually, depending on your needs.

Conclusion

Charging your crystals is a vital part of maintaining their effectiveness and ensuring that they continue to support your healing journey. Each method has its own unique qualities and can be chosen based on your preferences and the specific crystal you are working with. Whether you choose moonlight, sunlight, earth burial, sound, or energy healing, the key is to ensure that your crystal is regularly recharged to maintain its energetic potency. By incorporating these techniques into your crystal care routine, you help ensure that your stones stay vibrantly aligned with their healing properties and continue to support your intentions.

Clearing and Resetting Your Crystals

Crystals are powerful tools for healing and energy work, but like any energy system, they can accumulate negative or stagnant energy over time. This is particularly true if they are used frequently, passed between people, or exposed to heavy emotional or environmental influences. To ensure that your crystals remain effective and maintain their vibrational purity, it's important to regularly clear and reset their energy. Clearing removes unwanted energies, while resetting helps align the crystal's energy to its natural, optimal frequency. Here are some common and effective methods for clearing and resetting your crystals.

1. Smudging

Smudging is one of the oldest and most popular methods of clearing crystals. This involves using sacred herbs like sage, palo santo, or sweetgrass to cleanse a crystal of any negative energy. The smoke from the burning herbs is believed to purify the energy of the crystal, clearing away any stagnant or unwanted vibrations.

To smudge your crystals, light the smudge stick and pass your crystal through the smoke, allowing it to be fully enveloped. You can move the crystal through the smoke for several seconds to a few minutes, depending on the size of the stone and the level of clearing needed. Smudging is particularly useful for crystals that have been used frequently or in situations that may have exposed them to negative energies.

2. Running Water

Water is a natural cleanser, and running water can be used to clear and reset crystals. The flow of water is believed to carry away negative energy, leaving the crystal clear and revitalized. The method involves holding the crystal under a stream of water, ideally natural water like a river, stream, or creek. If natural running water is not available, tap water can be used, though it's generally better to avoid salty or chlorinated water.

Not all crystals are suitable for water cleansing, as some stones are porous and can be damaged by moisture. For example, selenite, halite, and some forms of calcite should not be exposed to water. Always research your crystal's properties before using this method.

3. Earth Burial

Burying a crystal in the earth allows it to reset its energy by reconnecting with the natural grounding forces of the planet. The earth is a powerful energy cleanser, and burying a crystal for a day or two will clear any accumulated negative energy. Simply dig a small hole in the ground and bury the crystal, ensuring it is well-covered. This method is best suited for grounding crystals like hematite, black tourmaline, and obsidian, which benefit from a deep connection with the earth.

After retrieving the crystal, it will feel reset and connected to the earth's natural energy. This method is particularly effective for restoring the energy of stones that have been used for protection or that have absorbed heavy energies.

4. Selenite Cleansing

Selenite is known for its cleansing and purifying properties, and it can be used to clear other crystals without direct contact with water or sunlight. Selenite is a high-vibration crystal that has the ability to absorb negative energy, leaving other crystals free of unwanted vibrations. Place your crystal on a selenite plate or near a selenite wand overnight to allow the energy transfer. The selenite will help reset the crystal's energy to its natural state.

This method is particularly effective for delicate crystals that may be damaged by water or sunlight, such as lapis lazuli, malachite, or amethyst. Selenite works gently and effectively, restoring the crystal's energetic balance without harm.

5. Sound and Vibration

Sound is another powerful tool for clearing crystals. The vibrations produced by sound waves can help dislodge and clear any stagnant or negative energy from a crystal, resetting it to its natural frequency. You can use tools like Tibetan singing bowls, tuning forks, or crystal sound bowls, which are tuned to specific frequencies that align with the crystal's energy.

To clear your crystal with sound, place it near the sound source and allow the vibrations to penetrate and energize the stone. For example, playing a singing bowl near the crystal will produce harmonic frequencies that help clear any accumulated energies. This method works particularly well with high-vibration stones like clear quartz, amethyst, and citrine.

6. Salt (Dry or Salt Water)

Salt is another traditional method of cleansing crystals. Salt has natural purifying properties, and it can help absorb negative energies from the crystal. There are two main methods for using salt:

- **Dry Salt:** For crystals that are safe to be in direct contact with salt (such as black tourmaline and clear quartz), you can bury them in a bowl of dry sea salt or

Himalayan pink salt for several hours or overnight. The salt absorbs any negativity, and the crystal will be recharged.
- **Salt Water:** For larger stones or those that require more intense cleansing, you can dissolve sea salt or Himalayan salt in water and place the crystal in the water for a short period. Be sure to check if the crystal is water-safe before using this method.

As with water cleansing, some crystals (like selenite, malachite, or pyrite) should not come into contact with salt or saltwater, as it can damage them.

7. Sunlight

Sunlight is a powerful source of energy and can be used to reset and charge your crystals. The sun's rays have the ability to invigorate and recharge crystals, especially those that are used for physical or energetic healing. Simply place your crystal in direct sunlight for a few hours or up to a full day, depending on the crystal's needs and tolerance.

However, be mindful that some crystals, like amethyst, rose quartz, and fluorite, can fade or lose their color when exposed to prolonged sunlight. For these crystals, it's better to limit their exposure to a few hours or to use other methods, such as moonlight or selenite.

8. Visualization

If you're unable to use physical methods of clearing or resetting, visualization can be an effective alternative. Sit quietly with your crystal in your hands and close your eyes. Imagine a bright, cleansing light surrounding the crystal, clearing away any negative energy. Visualize this light moving through the crystal, resetting it and aligning it with its natural, positive vibration.

This technique relies on the power of your intention and energy, making it an ideal choice when you are in a situation where other methods aren't feasible. Visualization can be particularly helpful for charging or resetting crystals during meditation or energy healing sessions.

9. Reiki and Energy Healing

Reiki, the Japanese healing technique that involves channeling energy, can also be used to clear and reset crystals. A trained Reiki practitioner can use their hands to direct energy into the crystal, clearing away negative energy and restoring balance. This method works by transferring healing energy from the practitioner to the crystal, allowing it to reset and align with its natural frequency.

Reiki works especially well with high-vibration crystals like clear quartz, amethyst, and labradorite, which benefit from the energetic boost.

Conclusion

Clearing and resetting your crystals is an essential part of working with them effectively. Regular cleansing ensures that they stay energetically pure and ready to assist with your healing, manifestation, or spiritual practices. Whether you choose smudging, water, earth burial, sound, or energy work, the key is to find the method that resonates with both you and your crystals. By maintaining your crystals' energetic health, you ensure that they continue to provide support and align with your personal energy, helping you achieve your goals and intentions.

Crystals in Your Environment

Crystals are not only tools for personal healing but can also play a significant role in enhancing the energy of your living or working environment. The vibrations of crystals interact with the space around them, creating an atmosphere that supports emotional, mental, and physical well-being. By strategically placing crystals throughout your environment, you can invite positive energy, promote harmony, and even improve the ambiance of your home or office. Here are some key ways to use crystals to transform your environment.

1. Promoting Calm and Relaxation

Certain crystals are known for their calming properties, making them ideal for creating a peaceful environment. For instance, amethyst, rose quartz, and lepidolite are well-suited for spaces where relaxation and emotional healing are the focus. Placing these crystals in your bedroom or meditation area can encourage restful sleep, stress relief, and emotional balance. Amethyst, in particular, is a highly effective crystal for promoting relaxation and spiritual awareness, while rose quartz is associated with unconditional love and healing, helping to create a nurturing, peaceful environment.

To enhance the effect, place these crystals on nightstands, shelves, or even under pillows to ensure that their calming energies are present as you sleep or unwind.

2. Purifying and Cleansing Energy

Crystals like selenite, black tourmaline, and clear quartz are excellent for purifying and clearing negative energy from your environment. Selenite, often considered a "self-cleansing" stone, can be placed in corners of rooms or near entryways to keep the space energetically clear. Black tourmaline is a powerful grounding stone known for its ability to absorb negative energy, making it a great choice for placing near doors, windows, or workspaces where stress or tension may accumulate. Clear quartz is versatile and amplifies the healing energy of other crystals, so it works well as a general purifier in any room.

By keeping your environment clear of negative energies, these stones can help ensure that only positive, harmonious energy remains, boosting the overall mood of the space.

3. Enhancing Focus and Productivity

For spaces where focus, concentration, and productivity are important, certain crystals can help enhance mental clarity and energy flow. Crystals like citrine, carnelian, and fluorite are known for their ability to stimulate creativity, improve focus, and energize the mind. Citrine is particularly effective in work environments because it is thought to promote success, abundance, and mental clarity. Carnelian, a stone of motivation, is ideal for creative spaces or home offices, as it encourages action and vitality. Fluorite helps organize thoughts and clear mental fog, making it great for study areas or places where decision-making takes place.

Placing these stones on desks, in study areas, or near workstations can support a productive, clear, and focused atmosphere.

4. Creating an Uplifting Atmosphere

If you're looking to bring more joy, positivity, and enthusiasm into your space, crystals like sunstone, citrine, and yellow jasper are excellent choices. These stones are all associated with the solar plexus chakra, which governs personal power, confidence, and motivation. Sunstone, with its radiant orange and gold tones, is known to encourage optimism and self-empowerment, while citrine, often referred to as the "merchant's stone," is believed to attract abundance and prosperity. Yellow jasper, another stone of optimism, works to balance and invigorate the energy of a room.

By placing these bright, energizing stones in high-traffic areas or communal spaces, you can foster an environment that feels uplifting, optimistic, and full of life.

5. Balancing the Energy of a Room

Crystals can also be used to balance the energy of a room or area where different types of energy might be at play. In spaces that feel chaotic or overly energetic, grounding stones like hematite, black tourmaline, or smoky quartz are ideal. These stones can be placed at the corners of a room or near entryways to absorb excess energy and create a calm, balanced atmosphere. Hematite, in particular, is known for its ability to help anchor energy, making it perfect for spaces that are prone to emotional intensity or overstimulation.

On the other hand, if a room feels stagnant or lacks vitality, you can use crystals like rose quartz, amethyst, or jade to bring in harmonious, loving energy. These stones work well in places where you want to encourage healing, peace, and positive interactions.

6. Improving Sleep Quality

To create an environment conducive to restful sleep, crystals like amethyst, lepidolite, and moonstone can be especially helpful. Amethyst has a soothing and calming energy that can help quiet the mind and promote deep, restful sleep, making it ideal for placing under pillows or on nightstands. Lepidolite, known for its calming and balancing properties, can reduce anxiety and promote emotional stability, helping you to unwind before bed. Moonstone, with its gentle energy, is associated with enhancing intuition and emotional clarity, making it perfect for a peaceful, dream-filled night.

If you're experiencing insomnia or disrupted sleep, placing these stones near your bed or on a bedside table can help restore tranquility and ensure a more restful, restorative sleep.

7. Improving Air Quality and Feng Shui

Crystals can also be used in conjunction with Feng Shui principles to enhance the energy flow of a space and improve air quality. According to Feng Shui, the placement of crystals in specific areas of the home can help promote harmony and balance. For example, clear quartz and amethyst can be placed in the center of the home or room to encourage balance, while black tourmaline is often placed near the door to ward off negative energy. Himalayan salt crystals, which are believed to improve air quality by releasing negative ions, can also be placed around the home or in office spaces to purify the air and reduce electromagnetic pollution.

8. Personal Spaces

In personal spaces like your bedroom or office, choosing crystals that align with your personal needs and intentions can significantly enhance your experience. If you're looking for protection, stones like black tourmaline or obsidian are excellent choices to ward off unwanted energies. For love and relationship energy, consider placing rose quartz or garnet in areas where you spend time with loved ones. If you want to invite abundance and prosperity, citrine and green aventurine can be placed in your office or business areas to attract success.

By intentionally placing crystals in the spaces where you spend the most time, you can create an environment that supports your emotional, mental, and spiritual growth.

Conclusion

The energy of your environment plays a crucial role in shaping your mood, productivity, and well-being. Crystals are an effective, natural way to enhance and transform the energy of any space, whether you're aiming for relaxation, focus, positivity, or healing. By understanding the unique properties of different crystals, you can strategically place them throughout your home or workplace to create an environment that supports your needs and intentions. With regular care and attention, your crystals can continue to amplify the energy around you, helping you live in a space filled with positive, vibrant energy.

Crystals have long been recognized for their ability to influence the energy of a space, and using them in the home and workplace can provide a wealth of benefits, from promoting emotional well-being to boosting productivity and creativity. By strategically placing different types of crystals throughout these environments, you can foster a positive, harmonious atmosphere that supports both personal and professional growth. Here's how to effectively incorporate crystals into your home and workplace.

1. Creating a Calm and Relaxing Home Environment

Many people seek tranquility and emotional balance in their homes, and certain crystals are particularly effective at promoting these qualities. Amethyst, for example, is well-known for its calming energy, which can help reduce stress and anxiety. It's ideal for bedrooms or meditation spaces, where relaxation is key. Placing amethyst near the bed or under a pillow can also enhance the quality of your sleep, as it encourages peaceful and restorative rest.

Rose quartz, the stone of unconditional love, is another excellent choice for the home, especially in living areas or places where family members gather. This crystal fosters love, compassion, and emotional healing, creating an environment where relationships can thrive. Its gentle, nurturing energy helps ease tension and promotes a sense of comfort and security.

For those seeking a more serene environment, lepidolite is an excellent option. Known for its ability to balance emotions and reduce anxiety, lepidolite works well in areas of the home where you need to unwind and disconnect from the stresses of daily life.

2. Boosting Productivity and Focus in the Workplace

In the workplace, the energy of your surroundings can significantly impact your level of focus, creativity, and productivity. Citrine, a bright yellow crystal associated with abundance and mental clarity, is often used to enhance these qualities. Its energy is invigorating and stimulating, making it ideal for desks, workstations, or areas where brainstorming and decision-making take place. Citrine is also believed to attract prosperity, making it a great addition to any business environment.

Fluorite, with its ability to help organize thoughts and clear mental fog, is another excellent choice for workplaces. It is particularly useful in settings where clear thinking and precision are required, such as offices or study areas. Placing fluorite on your desk can help you stay focused, organized, and clear-headed, improving your ability to manage tasks and deadlines.

For those looking for an energy boost to combat fatigue or mental blocks, carnelian is a powerful choice. Known for its ability to increase motivation, creativity, and physical energy, carnelian is perfect for creative spaces like studios or areas where innovation is important. Its vibrant, fiery energy can also help you overcome procrastination and stay on track with projects.

3. Encouraging Harmony and Collaboration in Group Settings

In environments where teamwork and collaboration are essential, such as in shared offices or meeting rooms, crystals that promote harmony, communication, and mutual respect can create a more cohesive and supportive atmosphere. Blue lace agate, for example, is a gentle stone that enhances communication and helps clear blockages in the throat chakra, making it ideal for facilitating open dialogue and understanding among team members.

Labradorite is another excellent choice for group settings, as it is believed to promote harmony and balance, while also encouraging creativity and new ideas. It's particularly helpful in workplaces where innovative thinking and problem-solving are central. Its energy helps prevent conflicts and fosters a cooperative environment, making it ideal for team meetings or brainstorming sessions.

4. Protection and Grounding in the Home and Workplace

Both the home and workplace can be susceptible to negative energies, whether from external sources or interpersonal dynamics. Certain crystals are particularly effective at protecting spaces and grounding energy. Black tourmaline, a powerful protective stone, is known for its ability to absorb negative energy and provide a sense of security and stability. Placing black tourmaline near doorways or windows helps to shield the space from unwanted influences, while also grounding any excess or erratic energy in the environment.

Hematite, another grounding stone, works by connecting the energy of the space to the earth. It is especially beneficial in environments where there is a lot of mental activity, as it can help reduce stress and encourage focus. Hematite can be placed in corners of the room or near workstations to create a calming, stabilizing influence.

In the home, especially in high-traffic areas or places where tensions may arise (like the kitchen or family room), you can also use shungite. Known for its ability to absorb electromagnetic radiation and negative energy, shungite can protect your space from harmful energies emitted by electronic devices.

5. Enhancing Emotional Well-Being in the Home

For a home that promotes emotional healing and balance, certain crystals can help create a nurturing and supportive environment. Moonstone, for instance, is a stone associated with intuition, emotional healing, and new beginnings. It's ideal for living rooms, bedrooms, or spaces where family members spend time together, as it encourages harmony and emotional connection. Moonstone's gentle, soothing energy can help ease emotional tension and support self-reflection.

Sodalite is another crystal that promotes emotional balance, especially when dealing with stress or anxiety. Its energy is calming and helps to release mental blockages, making it a good addition to spaces where personal reflection or relaxation is needed. Sodalite is also known to encourage rational thinking and decision-making, making it a beneficial stone for spaces where important discussions take place.

6. Creating an Inviting and Positive Atmosphere

In spaces where you want to encourage a sense of positivity and joy, certain crystals can lift the energy of the room and attract good vibes. Sunstone, a bright and uplifting crystal, is known for its ability to boost mood, encourage optimism, and promote personal empowerment. Its radiant energy can make any space feel more welcoming and lively. Place sunstone in entryways or living areas to invite positivity and vibrant energy into your home.

Clear quartz, often called the "master healer," is another excellent crystal for amplifying the energy of a space. Its clarity and ability to clear away negative energy makes it a versatile stone that can be used in any room to promote healing, clarity, and positivity. Clear quartz also amplifies the energies of other crystals, so it can be used in combination with other stones to strengthen their effects.

7. Use in Meditation and Relaxation Areas

If you have a dedicated space in your home or office for meditation, yoga, or relaxation, crystals can significantly enhance the atmosphere. Smoky quartz, known for its grounding properties, helps to deepen meditation and create a peaceful, relaxed environment. It aids in releasing negative emotions, making it ideal for spaces dedicated to emotional healing or deep thought.

Amethyst is also highly effective in meditation areas, as it promotes spiritual awareness and clarity. Its soothing energy encourages a deeper connection to the self, making it a great crystal for spiritual practices.

8. Caring for Crystals in the Home and Workplace

Once placed in the home or workplace, crystals should be regularly cleansed and recharged to maintain their effectiveness. Crystals can absorb negative energy over time, so it's important to clean and reset them using methods such as smudging, water (for water-safe crystals), or placing them in the sunlight or moonlight to restore their energy.

In addition, be mindful of where you place your crystals. They should be placed in locations that align with their energy and purpose. For example, avoid placing protective stones like black tourmaline in places where you want to encourage creativity, as it may dampen the energy needed for inspiration. Understanding the specific properties of each crystal will help you make the most of their presence in your environment.

Conclusion

Crystals offer a powerful way to influence and enhance the energy of the spaces where we live and work. Whether you're seeking to create a calm and relaxing atmosphere in your home, boost focus and creativity in the workplace, or protect and balance the energy in both, there's a crystal for every need. By thoughtfully selecting and placing crystals in your environment, you can harness their unique properties to improve well-being, productivity, and emotional balance, creating spaces that nurture and support you every day.

Crystals can enhance the energy of any space, including your garden, by promoting growth, balance, and harmony. Whether you're looking to create a peaceful oasis, attract abundance, or encourage spiritual growth, the right crystals can serve as powerful tools to amplify the natural energy around you. By selecting specific stones for your garden, you can align with nature's rhythms and infuse your outdoor space with healing vibrations.

1. Crystals for Plant Growth

Certain crystals are known to promote vitality and support plant growth, making them ideal additions to your garden. One of the most popular crystals for this purpose is **carnelian**. Known for its vibrant energy, carnelian is believed to stimulate creativity and action. When placed in the soil or near plants, carnelian is said to encourage robust growth and vitality, as it helps to enhance the life force energy of the plants.

Another great option is **aventurine**, particularly green aventurine, which is often linked to luck, abundance, and fertility. It is said to encourage the flourishing of plants and help them thrive in a garden setting. Placing aventurine near the base of plants or in the soil can support their growth, while also attracting good fortune.

Citrine, with its sunny yellow hue, is another crystal associated with abundance and prosperity. Placing citrine in your garden is thought to invite prosperity, success, and a bountiful harvest. Its energy is believed to attract positive vibrations, which in turn enhances the vitality of your plants.

2. Crystals for Grounding and Protection

For gardens that require grounding and protection from negative energies, **black tourmaline** is an excellent choice. Known for its ability to absorb and transform negative energy, black tourmaline can help create a secure and protected space. Placing black tourmaline at the boundaries of your garden or near areas where you seek balance will help clear any unwanted energy, ensuring that the space remains peaceful and energetically harmonious.

Hematite is another grounding stone that can be used to stabilize the energy of your garden. Hematite is believed to connect the energy of your garden to the Earth, helping to create a stable foundation for plants to grow. It can also assist in dispelling excess or chaotic energy from the environment, ensuring a calm and centered atmosphere.

3. Crystals for Harmony and Balance

Creating a harmonious environment in your garden is essential for promoting peace, tranquility, and a balanced flow of energy. **Rose quartz**, the stone of love, is an excellent choice for bringing loving energy to your outdoor space. It promotes feelings of peace and compassion, both for yourself and for the plants in your garden. Rose quartz can be placed near garden seating areas or tucked amongst plants to create a calm and nurturing atmosphere.

Amethyst, with its soothing violet energy, is another crystal that promotes balance and spiritual healing. In the garden, amethyst can enhance spiritual growth, encouraging clarity and emotional peace. It is particularly useful in areas where you meditate, reflect, or connect with nature on a deeper level. Amethyst can also promote a sense of inner peace, making it an excellent addition to gardens that serve as spaces for relaxation and introspection.

4. Crystals for Fertility and Abundance

If you're looking to attract abundance, both in terms of plants and overall prosperity, **jade** is a crystal that aligns well with these intentions. Known for its association with wealth, abundance, and fertility, jade is said to bring positive energy that promotes the growth of plants and encourages a fruitful harvest. It can also create an environment of prosperity and good fortune.

Green calcite is another powerful stone that aligns with abundance and fertility. Often used for its healing properties, green calcite can help create a fertile environment where your plants can grow freely and easily. It's particularly useful for encouraging new growth and can be placed near young or newly planted greenery to support their development.

5. Crystals for Spiritual Growth and Connection to Nature

For those who wish to deepen their connection to nature and spiritual growth, **clear quartz** is a versatile and powerful crystal. Known as the "master healer," clear quartz is believed to amplify the energy of any other stone it's paired with. It can be placed throughout the garden to raise the overall energy and help connect you to the natural world in a deeper way.

Moonstone is another excellent choice for enhancing spiritual growth in the garden. Associated with the moon and feminine energy, moonstone is said to enhance intuition and emotional clarity. It can help you align with the natural cycles of the earth, promoting a deeper understanding of the rhythms of life. Placing moonstone in a garden can create an atmosphere conducive to reflection, healing, and spiritual growth.

6. Crystals for Protection from Pests

If your garden struggles with pests or unwanted critters, certain crystals may help keep them at bay. **Amethyst** is sometimes used to deter pests, particularly those that are attracted to the energy of plants. Placing amethyst in strategic locations around your garden can create an energetic boundary that may prevent pests from entering.

Similarly, **obsidian** is a protective stone that can help keep unwanted energies and pests away. Obsidian's grounding energy helps protect the garden from negative influences, while its natural strength is thought to shield plants from external threats. Placing pieces of obsidian around the perimeter of your garden or near plant beds may help safeguard your crops.

7. Crystals for Enhancing Flowering and Fruit-Bearing

For gardens that focus on flowering or fruit-bearing plants, certain crystals are thought to encourage blooms and fruits. **Garnet**, for instance, is believed to encourage a bountiful harvest and promote the vibrant growth of flowers. It is also associated with vitality and passion, which can help energize your garden and encourage flowers and fruits to reach their full potential.

Tiger's eye is another stone known to boost energy and promote growth. It is thought to support the blossoming of flowers and fruits, especially when paired with the intention of creating a garden full of vibrant life. Placing tiger's eye near flower beds or fruit-bearing plants can encourage a flourishing garden that brings both beauty and nourishment.

8. Crystals for Clearing Negative Energy in the Garden

Sometimes, gardens can become energetically stagnant, especially if they are neglected or if negative emotions have accumulated in the space. Crystals like **selenite** are ideal for clearing any stagnant or negative energy. Selenite's cleansing properties make it perfect for resetting the energetic atmosphere of your garden. Simply placing selenite near entrances, gates, or in the corners of your garden can refresh the space and restore positive energy.

Conclusion

Integrating crystals into your garden can enhance the growth and well-being of your plants while also promoting positive energy, protection, and spiritual growth. Whether you're seeking to attract abundance, create a harmonious space, or deepen your connection with nature, the right crystals can help you manifest your intentions and infuse your garden with healing vibrations. By carefully selecting and placing crystals based on their properties, you can create a garden that not only nurtures your plants but also nurtures your body, mind, and spirit.

Incorporating crystals into your living or workspaces can bring powerful benefits, and one of the most effective ways to do so is by using them in alignment with the principles of Feng Shui. This ancient Chinese practice focuses on creating harmony, balance, and positive energy flow (known as *chi*) within an environment. Crystals, with their unique energetic properties, can enhance this flow, clear blockages, and promote physical, emotional, and spiritual well-being.

1. The Role of Crystals in Feng Shui

In Feng Shui, every space is divided into different zones, each representing specific aspects of life, such as wealth, love, health, and career. Crystals can be used to activate or enhance the energy in these areas. For example, placing certain crystals in the *wealth* corner (the far-left corner of your home or office when facing the door) can attract abundance, while other stones can be used to promote peace, love, and overall prosperity.

The energy of crystals is believed to interact with the environment by either amplifying positive energies or absorbing and neutralizing negative ones. Crystals such as clear quartz, amethyst, and rose quartz are often used in Feng Shui to enhance various areas of life. Choosing the right crystal and placing it in the right area is key to achieving the desired effect.

2. Crystals for Wealth and Prosperity

In the *wealth* zone of your home or office, crystals can help attract abundance and prosperity. **Citrine** is a crystal closely linked with wealth and financial success in Feng

Shui. Its bright, sunny energy encourages optimism, creativity, and a sense of abundance. Placing citrine in the *wealth* corner or on your desk can activate this area, bringing positive financial energy into your life.

Pyrite, often referred to as 'fool's gold," is another crystal that is considered a powerful symbol of wealth and good fortune. In Feng Shui, it is placed in the *wealth* or *career* zones to attract financial opportunities. Its metallic luster represents the energy of abundance and success, making it an ideal stone for those looking to boost their income or career prospects.

Jade, a stone that represents prosperity, growth, and good luck, is also highly favored in Feng Shui. Its green color aligns with the energy of growth and fertility, making it ideal for promoting abundance in all areas of life, including wealth. Jade is commonly placed in areas where financial or material goals are pursued.

3. Crystals for Love and Relationships

The *love* corner of your home, located in the far-right corner when facing the door, is the area associated with relationships, marriage, and harmony. **Rose quartz** is the quintessential crystal for love in Feng Shui. Its gentle pink energy fosters compassion, emotional healing, and unconditional love, making it perfect for enhancing relationships, whether with a partner, family, or friends.

Amethyst also holds a special place in the Feng Shui practice for love, as it helps clear emotional blockages and promotes deep connection and understanding in relationships. It enhances spiritual energy, which can lead to greater emotional and relational harmony. Placing amethyst in the love zone helps create an atmosphere of mutual respect and open communication.

Garnet, a deep red stone, is another excellent choice for the love corner. It is said to promote passion, commitment, and vitality in romantic relationships. Its stimulating energy can help invigorate existing relationships and attract new love into your life.

4. Crystals for Health and Well-Being

The *health* area in Feng Shui is located in the center of the home or room, representing the overall balance of the body and mind. To promote vitality, healing, and well-being, **green aventurine** is often used. Known as the stone of luck and opportunity, aventurine can also help to balance energy and stimulate healing in the body. Placing it in the center of your living space can encourage good health and vitality for all inhabitants.

Clear quartz is another powerful crystal used in Feng Shui to enhance the energy of the health area. Its purifying and amplifying properties help maintain clear and positive energy flow throughout the body and environment, which supports mental and physical wellness.

Amethyst also plays a role in healing and overall well-being. Its calming energy helps to relieve stress, soothe anxiety, and promote a peaceful environment, aiding in the restoration of both emotional and physical health. Its purple hue is particularly effective in promoting mental clarity and emotional balance.

5. Crystals for Career and Success

The *career* area, which is located in the center-back section of a room or home, corresponds to your professional life, ambitions, and overall life path. **Black tourmaline** is a powerful grounding crystal that is often used in Feng Shui to protect and stabilize the energy in the career zone. It can help to absorb negative energy and provide a sense of security, enabling individuals to focus on their career goals with confidence.

Tiger's eye is also used in the career zone to promote courage, confidence, and focus. It's particularly effective in helping individuals overcome obstacles and stay motivated on their career path. The stone's golden-brown bands are associated with clarity and grounded decision-making, which can enhance your ability to achieve success in your professional endeavors.

Aventurine (specifically green aventurine) is another stone tied to success and opportunity. It's especially beneficial for those seeking new career opportunities or wanting to make significant progress in their professional life. Placing aventurine in the career area invites new opportunities and career growth.

6. Crystals for Clarity and Focus

To enhance clarity, focus, and mental sharpness in any space, **fluorite** is an excellent choice. Often referred to as the "genius stone," fluorite is believed to improve mental clarity, decision-making, and focus. In Feng Shui, it can be placed in areas where work or study takes place to enhance concentration and intellectual ability.

Lapis lazuli is another stone known for stimulating mental clarity and helping to open up the third eye chakra. Its deep blue energy supports truth, wisdom, and clear communication, making it a great addition to spaces where clear thinking and understanding are essential.

7. Crystals for Spirituality and Meditation

For promoting spiritual growth and a deeper connection to the universe, **amethyst** is widely used in Feng Shui. Its high-vibrational energy aligns with the crown chakra and encourages meditation, introspection, and higher states of consciousness. It's perfect for spaces dedicated to spiritual practices or areas where you seek peace and inner clarity.

Selenite, known for its cleansing and purifying properties, is also commonly used to enhance spiritual energy. It's believed to help clear negative or stagnant energy from a space, creating a peaceful, tranquil environment that is conducive to spiritual practice and deep meditation.

Clear quartz is another excellent choice for spiritual growth. As an amplifier of energy, clear quartz can enhance any spiritual practices you engage in, from meditation to prayer. Its ability to absorb and purify energy makes it ideal for clearing the space and elevating the overall vibration of your environment.

8. Crystals for Protection

In addition to promoting various aspects of life, crystals can also be used for protection, especially in areas that are more vulnerable to negative energy or external influences. **Black obsidian** is one of the strongest protective stones, and it can absorb and shield you from negative energies. It's commonly placed near entrances or in vulnerable corners of the home to create a protective barrier.

Hematite, with its grounding and protective properties, is another excellent stone for safeguarding your space. Its energy helps to stabilize your environment and provides a sense of security and protection from unwanted influences.

Conclusion

Using crystals in Feng Shui allows you to harmonize your living or work environment with the energy you wish to attract. By placing specific crystals in targeted areas of your home, you can enhance wealth, love, health, success, and spiritual growth while creating a balanced, positive space. Whether you're seeking clarity, abundance, or protection, the right crystal can amplify the energy of your space, bringing about a greater sense of well-being and purpose in your life.

Crystals can be a wonderful addition to the lives of children and animals, offering gentle healing energy and support for emotional, physical, and spiritual well-being. When used appropriately, these natural stones can help create a peaceful environment, promote relaxation, and encourage healing in both children and pets. Understanding the properties of various crystals and how to use them safely is essential when introducing them into the lives of young ones and animals.

1. Crystals for Children

Children are naturally sensitive to energies, and crystals can support their emotional growth and development in a nurturing and non-invasive way. Certain stones are particularly suited for addressing the unique needs of children, such as calming anxiety, boosting self-esteem, or promoting restful sleep.

Amethyst is an excellent crystal for children, especially those who struggle with sleep disturbances or nightmares. Its soothing, calming energy can promote a sense of peace and tranquility, making it a great addition to a child's bedroom. Amethyst is also known to support emotional balance and spiritual growth, helping children process their feelings and develop their intuition.

Rose quartz is another stone that works well with children. Known as the stone of unconditional love, rose quartz promotes emotional healing, compassion, and positive self-esteem. It can help children feel safe and loved, which is particularly helpful for those experiencing feelings of fear, loneliness, or sadness. Placing rose quartz under a pillow or on a nightstand can create a calming energy in the room, fostering a loving environment for rest and emotional well-being.

Citrine is a joyful and uplifting crystal that encourages positivity and self-confidence. For children who need a boost in their personal strength or who struggle with self-doubt, citrine can help to enhance their self-esteem and encourage a positive outlook on life. Its sunny energy is also beneficial for reducing stress and promoting motivation, making it an excellent choice for children who are facing academic or social challenges.

Selenite is known for its cleansing properties, and it is particularly useful for children who may be sensitive to negative energies or overstimulation. Selenite's calming and purifying energy helps to clear away any emotional clutter or negativity, promoting mental clarity and a peaceful state of mind. It can be placed in a child's room to create a tranquil and harmonious space.

Lepidolite, with its lithium content, is often recommended for children who experience anxiety, stress, or emotional imbalances. This soothing stone can help ease tension and stabilize mood swings, offering emotional support during times of upheaval or change. It is also helpful in fostering restful sleep, making it ideal for children who are restless at night.

2. Crystals for Animals

Just like children, animals can also benefit from the healing properties of crystals. Crystals can help pets recover from illness, relieve anxiety, and even support their overall health and vitality. However, when using crystals for animals, it is essential to approach it with care and mindfulness, ensuring that the crystals are safe and that they are placed in a manner that is comfortable for the animal.

Amethyst is not only helpful for children but also for pets. Its calming and soothing properties are beneficial for animals who experience stress, anxiety, or fear. Amethyst can help create a tranquil environment, making it ideal for pets who may be frightened by loud noises, changes in routine, or travel. Amethyst can be placed near the pet's bed or favorite resting spot to promote relaxation and alleviate anxiety.

Rose quartz is also a great choice for pets, particularly for those who are emotionally sensitive or have experienced trauma. It promotes unconditional love and emotional healing, helping animals to feel more secure and loved. Rose quartz can assist in strengthening the bond between the pet and its owner, fostering a deep connection built on trust and affection. It can be placed near the pet's sleeping area or even worn as a pendant by the pet if they are comfortable with it.

Black tourmaline is a protective stone that helps to shield animals from negative or overwhelming energies. If a pet is experiencing fear, restlessness, or aggression, black tourmaline can provide grounding and a sense of security. It absorbs negative energy and helps to create a calm, safe environment. This stone is also excellent for pets who are exposed to environmental stressors, such as loud noises or unfamiliar surroundings.

Clear quartz is a versatile and powerful crystal that can benefit both children and animals. Known for its ability to amplify energy, clear quartz can be used to cleanse and balance an animal's energy field. It can help with healing, emotional balance, and overall well-being. Clear quartz can be placed near a pet's bed or incorporated into their environment to create a healing, harmonious atmosphere.

Carnelian is a crystal that boosts vitality, energy, and confidence. For animals who are recovering from illness, surgery, or emotional trauma, carnelian can support healing and help restore energy. It also promotes a sense of enthusiasm and motivation, making it ideal for pets who need a little extra encouragement to engage in play or exercise.

Aventurine, especially green aventurine, is known for promoting physical healing and vitality, making it beneficial for animals recovering from injury or illness. This stone is also associated with abundance and prosperity, helping to create a positive and nurturing environment for pets. Aventurine can also support animals in overcoming fears and building confidence.

3. How to Use Crystals for Children and Animals

When using crystals for children or animals, it is essential to take a gentle approach. Here are some simple ways to incorporate crystals into their lives:

- **Crystal Placement**: Place crystals under pillows, in the corners of rooms, or near a child's or pet's sleeping area. This can create a peaceful and supportive environment for rest.
- **Crystal Jewelry**: For children and animals that are comfortable with wearing crystals, you can create a necklace or bracelet with crystal beads. Make sure the crystal is non-toxic and safe for prolonged contact.
- **Crystal Elixirs**: You can create crystal-infused water by placing a cleansed crystal in a glass of water (ensure the crystal is safe for water infusion). Offer this water to your child or pet for gentle healing. Always check that the crystal is non-toxic before using it this way.
- **Crystal Grids**: If your child or pet is open to it, create a crystal grid in their room or area. This involves arranging crystals in a specific pattern that corresponds to the intention you wish to set. For example, use calming stones like amethyst and rose quartz in a grid designed to promote relaxation.
- **Direct Contact**: For children, holding or playing with the crystals can be a tactile way to connect with their energy. For pets, place crystals near them during rest or play. Always observe your pet's response to ensure they are comfortable with the crystal.

4. Safety Considerations

When using crystals with children or pets, safety should be a top priority. Crystals should be kept out of reach of very young children, as they could be a choking hazard. For pets, ensure that the crystals are not small enough to be swallowed. Always choose polished stones, as rough or sharp crystals may pose a risk of injury. Additionally, make sure to regularly cleanse and recharge the crystals to maintain their optimal energy.

Conclusion

Crystals can be a powerful, supportive tool for both children and animals, providing emotional comfort, physical healing, and spiritual balance. By choosing the right crystals for specific needs and using them with care and intention, you can create a healing environment that promotes well-being, calm, and love for your loved ones—whether they are human or animal.

When selecting crystals for children, it's important to choose stones that are gentle, soothing, and safe for young energy. Crystals can support children emotionally, spiritually, and even physically, helping them navigate challenging feelings or experiences. By understanding the properties of different crystals and their effects, parents and caregivers can select those most beneficial for a child's specific needs.

1. Amethyst for Calm and Sleep

Amethyst is a calming stone with gentle, soothing energy, making it an excellent choice for children who struggle with anxiety, sleeplessness, or nightmares. The crystal's purifying energy promotes relaxation and emotional balance. Amethyst also enhances intuitive abilities, so it can be useful for children who are developing sensitivity or are highly intuitive. Placing amethyst near a child's bed or under their pillow can help them sleep peacefully and feel emotionally grounded.

2. Rose Quartz for Love and Compassion

Known as the stone of unconditional love, rose quartz is a nurturing and gentle crystal that can help children develop positive self-esteem and build harmonious relationships. This pink-hued stone supports emotional healing and creates a loving, compassionate energy, helping children who may be struggling with feelings of fear, sadness, or isolation. Rose quartz encourages empathy and emotional intelligence, making it a valuable tool for fostering kindness and love in the home. It can be placed under pillows, in a child's room, or even carried as a pocket stone.

3. Citrine for Confidence and Joy

Citrine is a vibrant yellow crystal that radiates positivity and joy. It's known to boost confidence, creativity, and personal power—qualities that can be particularly helpful for children who are shy, uncertain, or facing challenges with self-esteem. Citrine encourages a positive mindset and can be especially useful for children who need a little extra motivation or inspiration. It is also linked to the solar plexus chakra, the center of willpower and confidence. Citrine can be placed in the child's study area to encourage focus and a positive outlook on learning.

4. Clear Quartz for Amplifying Energy

Clear quartz is one of the most versatile and powerful crystals available. It is often referred to as a "master healer" because it amplifies energy and enhances the properties of other crystals. For children, clear quartz can help with mental clarity, concentration, and emotional balance. It can be used to support a child's overall well-being, whether they are studying, playing, or dealing with emotional challenges. Clear quartz can also be used to clear negative energies in a space, promoting a calm and harmonious environment.

5. Lepidolite for Emotional Balance

Lepidolite is a calming crystal that contains lithium, a substance known for its mood-stabilizing properties. This stone is especially helpful for children who may experience mood swings, anxiety, or emotional overload. Lepidolite helps bring emotional balance, calm, and a sense of peace. It is also beneficial for children dealing with stress, such as those experiencing changes in their lives (e.g., moving, new siblings, or school-related stress). Lepidolite can be placed in a child's room or carried as a small pendant to provide comfort and stability.

6. Black Tourmaline for Protection

Black tourmaline is a protective stone that helps guard against negative energies, electromagnetic radiation, and stress. For children who may be sensitive to external stimuli or who experience fear or anxiety, black tourmaline can help create a safe, grounded environment. It is an excellent stone for protecting children during times of change or when they need to feel secure in their surroundings. Black tourmaline can be placed near electronic devices, in bedrooms, or worn as jewelry to shield from negative energy and enhance feelings of safety.

7. Fluorite for Mental Clarity and Focus

Fluorite is a stone of mental clarity and focus, making it an excellent choice for children who need help with concentration, studying, or schoolwork. It is known to enhance learning abilities and clear mental fog. Fluorite's calming energy also reduces stress and anxiety, helping children to remain calm and collected when facing academic challenges or tests. This crystal can be placed in a study area or worn as jewelry to help boost concentration and clarity.

8. Selenite for Spiritual Cleansing

Selenite is a powerful cleansing stone that can purify and charge the energy of other crystals. It is also known for its ability to clear negative energy and create a peaceful environment. For children, selenite can help with emotional clarity and create a serene atmosphere. It's especially useful in spaces where children may feel overwhelmed or overstimulated. Selenite is ideal for purifying a child's room before sleep, ensuring that the space is clear of any negative or disruptive energy.

9. Aventurine for Growth and Healing

Green aventurine is a stone of growth, healing, and good fortune. This stone is perfect for children who need support in developing self-confidence or who are recovering from an illness or emotional difficulty. Aventurine is linked to the heart chakra, promoting healing and emotional balance, especially for children who may be feeling vulnerable or struggling with self-worth. It's also helpful in encouraging new beginnings and opportunities, making it a great stone for children facing transitions or new experiences, such as starting a new school or making new friends.

10. Carnelian for Motivation and Vitality

Carnelian is a warm, energizing crystal that stimulates motivation, vitality, and personal power. It can be particularly helpful for children who lack motivation, struggle with focus, or need a boost in energy. Carnelian encourages creativity, curiosity, and self-expression, helping children feel confident in exploring new activities or pursuing their passions. This crystal is also helpful in enhancing physical energy and vitality, making it a great choice for active children or those recovering from illness. Placing carnelian in a child's play area or near their creative space can encourage physical and mental vitality.

Safety Tips When Using Crystals for Children

- **Size and Shape**: Choose crystals that are large enough that they cannot be swallowed. Avoid sharp or jagged stones, as these can pose a safety hazard.
- **Avoid Small Crystals**: Small crystals can be a choking hazard, so avoid using crystals that could be easily ingested by young children.
- **Supervision**: Always supervise children when they are using or handling crystals, especially if they are new to crystal healing.
- **Cleansing Crystals**: Regularly cleanse and recharge crystals to maintain their positive energy. Crystals can absorb negative energies, so it's important to keep them energetically clear for your child's benefit.

Conclusion

Choosing the right crystals for children can enhance their emotional and physical well-being, promoting balance, love, and positive energy. By selecting gentle stones that support healing and growth, you can create an environment that nurtures your child's emotional health and spiritual development. Whether it's calming anxiety, boosting self-esteem, or encouraging creativity, crystals can be a wonderful tool to help children thrive.

Crystal Healing Techniques for Pets

Using crystals for pets can be a gentle and effective way to support their emotional, physical, and energetic well-being. Animals, like humans, can experience stress, anxiety, and illness, and crystals offer a natural, non-invasive method to help restore balance and promote healing. Understanding how to use crystals safely and effectively for pets is key to ensuring they receive the benefits of crystal healing without causing any discomfort or harm.

1. Understanding Pet Sensitivity to Energy

Pets, especially animals like dogs and cats, are highly sensitive to energy. They can pick up on the emotional states of their owners, as well as environmental energies, including negative or disruptive vibrations. This sensitivity makes them ideal candidates for the healing properties of crystals, as these stones can help clear negative energy, calm anxiety, and support physical healing.

Crystals work by interacting with the subtle energy field of the body, known as the aura or energy field. Each crystal has a unique vibration and frequency that can either balance, amplify, or soothe the energy around an animal. When used properly, crystals can help alleviate stress, promote relaxation, and support overall health.

2. Choosing the Right Crystals for Pets

Different crystals offer different benefits, so it's important to choose the right ones depending on the pet's needs. Here are some popular options:

- **Amethyst**: Known for its calming and healing properties, amethyst is perfect for pets that suffer from anxiety, fear, or hyperactivity. This crystal can help ease nervousness, promote relaxation, and support restful sleep. It's especially useful for pets that experience separation anxiety, travel stress, or restlessness.
- **Rose Quartz**: Often referred to as the stone of unconditional love, rose quartz is ideal for pets that need emotional healing, especially after trauma or neglect. It helps to promote a sense of safety, comfort, and affection, which can be helpful for animals who have experienced abandonment, abuse, or emotional distress.
- **Black Tourmaline**: This powerful protective stone helps to shield pets from negative energies, electromagnetic radiation, and stress. Black tourmaline can be used to create a safe, grounding environment for pets who are highly sensitive or

easily overstimulated. It can also be helpful for pets that are fearful, anxious, or exhibiting signs of aggression.
- **Clear Quartz**: Clear quartz is a versatile crystal that can be used to amplify the energy of other crystals or cleanse the energy in an environment. It can be particularly helpful for pets recovering from illness, as it supports healing and balances the energy in their body. Clear quartz can also help promote mental clarity and relaxation.
- **Citrine**: Known for its uplifting energy, citrine is ideal for pets who need a boost in vitality, motivation, or mood. It's also beneficial for pets who are recovering from illness or surgery, as it encourages vitality and a positive outlook. Citrine's energizing properties can help pets feel more active and engaged.
- **Selenite**: Selenite is a purifying crystal that helps to clear negative energy and promote a sense of peace. It's ideal for creating a calming environment for pets, especially in situations where they may feel stressed or overwhelmed, such as during thunderstorms, fireworks, or travel.
- **Hematite**: Hematite is known for its grounding and stabilizing properties. This crystal is beneficial for pets that feel out of balance or disoriented, particularly if they are recovering from physical injuries or illnesses. Hematite helps to bring stability to the body and energy field, promoting strength and resilience.

3. How to Use Crystals with Pets

There are several ways to incorporate crystals into your pet's life. Each method can be tailored to the specific needs of your animal:

Crystal Placement

One of the simplest ways to use crystals with pets is by placing them in their environment. For example, place a calming crystal like amethyst or rose quartz near their bed, in their favorite resting spot, or on their collar. This allows the crystal to interact with the animal's energy field passively throughout the day or night.

Crystal Jewelry for Pets

Some pets may be comfortable wearing crystal jewelry, such as a collar adorned with crystal beads or a pendant. When using crystals in this way, make sure the crystals are securely attached to the collar or harness and that they are large enough that they cannot be swallowed. Crystals like rose quartz, amethyst, or black tourmaline can be worn as pendants to provide ongoing support throughout the day.

Crystal Elixirs

Another way to introduce crystals into a pet's routine is by creating crystal-infused water. To make a crystal elixir, place a clean, polished crystal (make sure it is safe for water infusion) in a glass or bowl of water for several hours. Once the energy from the crystal has been infused into the water, you can offer it to your pet. Be sure to remove the crystal from the water before allowing the pet to drink, and only use non-toxic crystals. Some pet owners also place the infused water near the pet's food or water bowl to encourage healing and balance.

Crystal Grids

For pets dealing with emotional or physical issues, you can create a crystal grid in their space. This involves arranging specific crystals in a pattern that corresponds to a particular healing intention. For example, a grid using amethyst, rose quartz, and black tourmaline can help calm a pet's anxiety while promoting emotional healing. You can place the grid near your pet's resting area or simply keep it in a quiet, private space.

Direct Contact with Crystals

Some pets may be receptive to direct contact with crystals. Gently placing a crystal on or near your pet's body can help facilitate energy healing. For pets that are not comfortable with direct touch, simply placing the crystal nearby may still be effective. For example, placing a piece of rose quartz near a cat's sleeping area can encourage a sense of calm and comfort, while a piece of hematite can be used to stabilize energy for an active dog.

4. Signs That Crystals Are Helping Your Pet

After introducing crystals into your pet's environment or routine, you may start to notice positive changes in their behavior and well-being. These changes can include:

- A noticeable decrease in anxiety or stress
- Improved sleep patterns or relaxation
- Enhanced physical vitality or recovery from illness or surgery
- A calmer, more balanced demeanor
- A stronger bond with their human family members

It's important to monitor your pet's response to the crystals, as every animal may react differently. If your pet shows signs of discomfort or unease, discontinue use or try a different crystal.

5. Safety Considerations

While crystals are generally safe for pets, there are some important precautions to keep in mind:

- **Avoid Small Crystals**: Crystals that are too small can pose a choking hazard for pets, especially dogs and cats that may chew on them. Always use larger crystals or ensure that smaller stones are kept out of reach.
- **Check for Toxicity**: Some crystals are toxic if ingested. Always ensure that the crystals you use are safe for pets. Avoid using crystals that may crumble or break into sharp pieces that could cause injury.
- **Monitor Pet's Comfort**: Not all pets will respond positively to the presence of crystals. If your pet shows signs of discomfort, such as restlessness or avoidance, remove the crystal and observe their behavior.

6. Conclusion

Crystals can be a powerful and natural tool for promoting emotional and physical healing in pets. By choosing the right crystals and using them safely, you can help your pet experience reduced stress, enhanced relaxation, and improved overall health. Whether through crystal placement, jewelry, elixirs, or direct contact, crystals offer a gentle, non-invasive way to support your pet's well-being. Always observe your pet's response and consult a veterinarian if you have concerns about their health or behavior.

Safety and Precautions when Using Crystals with Children and Animals

Using crystals for healing can be a beneficial practice for both children and animals, offering emotional, physical, and energetic support. However, it's important to take safety precautions to ensure that the crystals are used appropriately and do not pose any risks. Children and animals are especially sensitive to their environment and the energy around them, so understanding the best practices when incorporating crystals into their lives is essential.

1. Choosing the Right Crystals

When selecting crystals for children or animals, it's important to choose stones that are safe, gentle, and appropriate for their needs. Some crystals are not suitable for direct contact with children or pets due to their chemical composition, fragility, or sharp edges.

- **Non-toxic Crystals**: Always ensure that the crystals you choose are safe for both children and animals. Some crystals, such as those containing lead, arsenic, or other toxic elements, should be avoided. Crystals like amethyst, rose quartz, clear quartz, and selenite are generally safe, while stones like malachite, galena, or turquoise can be toxic if ingested.
- **Size Considerations**: Crystals should be large enough to avoid the risk of choking or ingestion, especially for young children or small animals. Small, sharp, or fragile crystals can break into pieces, creating a potential hazard. Choose smooth, large, tumbled stones or polished crystals that are less likely to cause injury.
- **Avoid Crystals That Crumble**: Some crystals, such as selenite, can crumble or break easily. If you're using crystals with pets or children, avoid those that can shatter into small, sharp pieces, which could lead to injury if ingested or stepped on.

2. Supervision is Key

Children and pets are naturally curious, and they may be drawn to crystals because of their colors, textures, and energy. As such, it's important to supervise them closely whenever crystals are in use, particularly with small children or animals that might try to chew or swallow them.

- **Supervise Handling**: Always supervise your child or pet when they are handling or interacting with crystals, especially if they are new to the practice. Even if the crystals are large and non-toxic, children and pets may be tempted to play with them or place them in their mouths.
- **Limit Access for Very Young Children**: For babies or toddlers who are still in the phase of putting objects in their mouths, avoid leaving crystals within their reach. Small crystals or stones with sharp edges can be a choking hazard, so it's best to only allow these objects under adult supervision.
- **Monitor Pets Closely**: Animals, particularly those that chew or nibble on things, should be monitored closely around crystals. Even non-toxic crystals can be dangerous if they are ingested in large quantities, and small shards could cause harm to your pet's digestive system or mouth.

3. Cleansing Crystals Regularly

Crystals absorb energy from their surroundings, including both positive and negative energies. Over time, this can result in the buildup of unwanted or stagnant energy, which could affect their effectiveness and possibly create discomfort for children or animals. Regularly cleansing your crystals helps to maintain their purity and vitality.

- **Safe Cleansing Methods**: There are various ways to cleanse crystals, but some methods may not be suitable for use around children or pets. For example, using salt or harsh chemicals can damage certain stones and should be avoided. Safe methods for cleansing crystals include using water (for water-safe stones), smudging with sage or palo santo, placing them in moonlight, or using sound vibration (such as a singing bowl).
- **Cleansing the Environment**: Just as crystals absorb energy, they can also influence the energy of the environment around them. Regularly clear the space where your child or pet spends time to ensure the energy remains positive and balanced.

4. Avoid Overloading with Crystals

While crystals can be beneficial, they should be used in moderation, especially when working with children or pets. Too many crystals in close proximity could overwhelm their energy field, leading to overstimulation or agitation.

- **Start Slowly**: Introduce crystals one at a time, particularly when you're using them with children or pets for the first time. This allows you to observe how they respond to the crystal's energy and make adjustments if needed.
- **Energy Sensitivity**: Children, in particular, may be more sensitive to the energy of crystals due to their developing energy systems. Start with gentle stones like rose quartz or amethyst and watch for signs of comfort or discomfort. If a child seems

restless or overly energetic, it could be a sign that they're reacting to the energy of the crystal.

5. Avoid Using Crystals on the Skin for Sensitive Individuals

While many people enjoy wearing crystals as jewelry or carrying them in their pockets, this might not be suitable for everyone, particularly for children and animals with sensitive skin. Some crystals, especially those with sharp edges or rough textures, can irritate the skin if placed directly on the body.

- **Use Crystals as Environmental Tools**: Instead of placing crystals directly on the body of a child or pet, consider using them in the surrounding environment. Placing crystals on shelves, under the bed, or in specific areas of the home can still provide their energetic benefits without direct contact.
- **Crystal Jewelry for Children and Pets**: If you choose to use crystal jewelry with children or pets, ensure that the jewelry is securely attached and made of durable materials. Avoid using small beads or delicate chains that could break or be ingested.

6. Choosing Appropriate Crystals for Children and Pets

Certain crystals may be more beneficial or appropriate for children and pets based on their calming, protective, or healing properties. Some of the best options include:

- **Amethyst**: Calms anxiety and promotes restful sleep.
- **Rose Quartz**: Encourages love, healing, and emotional balance.
- **Citrine**: Boosts positivity and self-esteem.
- **Black Tourmaline**: Provides protection from negative energies and electromagnetic fields.
- **Clear Quartz**: Supports overall healing and amplifies energy.
- **Selenite**: Cleanses and purifies the environment.

However, certain crystals, such as those with toxic properties (e.g., malachite, galena, or turquoise), should be avoided in environments with children or pets. Always research a crystal's properties before introducing it into your space.

7. Signs of Discomfort or Negative Reactions

Both children and animals are highly sensitive to energies, and it's important to observe any changes in behavior when crystals are introduced. Signs that a child or pet may not be comfortable with a particular crystal or the energy it emits include:

- **Restlessness or Irritability**: If a child becomes unusually fussy or agitated when near a crystal, it might not be the right fit for them.

- **Avoidance Behavior**: Animals may shy away from crystals, particularly if they are placed in areas where the animal spends a lot of time.
- **Physical Symptoms**: Any signs of physical discomfort, such as pawing at the crystal, licking or chewing it, or exhibiting signs of distress, should be taken seriously.

If any of these signs occur, remove the crystal from the area immediately and reassess whether it's the right choice for your child or pet.

8. Conclusion

Crystals can be a powerful tool for enhancing well-being, but when working with children and animals, it's essential to use them with caution and mindfulness. By choosing the right crystals, ensuring they are safe and non-toxic, and monitoring their use, you can help create a positive environment that supports healing, balance, and comfort. Always observe how your child or pet responds, and be prepared to adjust your approach based on their unique needs. With care and attention, crystals can become a valuable addition to your home, offering gentle healing for both children and animals.

Crystals for Personal Growth

Personal growth is a continuous journey of self-discovery, transformation, and empowerment. Crystals, with their unique energetic properties, have long been used as tools to support individuals on this path. By interacting with the energy fields of our bodies and minds, crystals can help clear blockages, enhance emotional balance, and foster a deeper connection with our inner selves. Each crystal carries a vibration that resonates with different aspects of personal growth, from improving self-esteem to enhancing creativity and fostering emotional healing.

1. Crystals for Self-Awareness

Self-awareness is a cornerstone of personal growth. It involves gaining insight into your thoughts, emotions, and behaviors, and understanding how they influence your life. Crystals that support self-reflection and heightened awareness can be invaluable on this journey.

- **Amethyst**: This crystal is widely known for its ability to calm the mind and encourage deep reflection. Amethyst enhances mental clarity, making it easier to assess your true desires and motivations. It promotes a sense of inner peace, helping you to quiet distractions and focus on what truly matters in your life.
- **Labradorite**: Known as the "stone of transformation," labradorite encourages deep personal change and helps you tap into your inner wisdom. This stone can awaken your intuitive abilities and strengthen your connection to your higher self, allowing for clearer insight into your life's purpose.

2. Crystals for Emotional Healing

Emotional growth is just as vital as mental and spiritual growth. Crystals that support emotional healing can help you process past traumas, release negative emotions, and cultivate a more positive outlook.

- **Rose Quartz**: The quintessential stone for love and emotional healing, rose quartz promotes self-love, compassion, and forgiveness. It helps to open the heart chakra, allowing you to heal from past emotional wounds and embrace unconditional love for yourself and others. This crystal encourages a deep connection with your emotional self, fostering acceptance and understanding.

- **Moonstone**: Associated with the divine feminine and the cycles of the moon, moonstone enhances emotional balance and intuition. It helps you to navigate periods of emotional flux and encourages a sense of peace during times of change or uncertainty. Moonstone is particularly beneficial for those who are working through emotional patterns related to the past or unresolved feelings.

3. Crystals for Confidence and Self-Esteem

Confidence is essential for personal growth, as it allows you to step into your power and pursue your goals with conviction. Crystals that support self-esteem can help you overcome self-doubt and recognize your intrinsic worth.

- **Citrine**: This bright, vibrant crystal is known for its ability to boost self-confidence and promote positivity. Citrine encourages a sense of abundance and personal power, making it ideal for overcoming limiting beliefs and stepping into a more confident version of yourself. It also helps to dispel negative energy and replace it with a more optimistic mindset.
- **Tiger's Eye**: A powerful grounding and protection stone, tiger's eye enhances courage and strength. It supports you in making decisions with clarity and confidence, especially in moments of self-doubt or uncertainty. Tiger's eye fosters inner stability and helps you trust in your ability to navigate challenges.

4. Crystals for Manifestation and Goal Setting

Personal growth is closely tied to setting and achieving goals. Crystals that promote manifestation can help you stay focused, clear, and motivated as you work toward your dreams.

- **Clear Quartz**: Often called the "master healer," clear quartz amplifies the energy of other crystals and supports clarity of thought. It enhances your ability to visualize and manifest your desires by aligning your energy with your intentions. Clear quartz can help you stay focused on your goals and ensure that your energy is directed toward achieving them.
- **Green Aventurine**: Known as the "stone of opportunity," green aventurine is a powerful crystal for attracting luck and abundance. It promotes confidence in pursuing new opportunities and helps you take inspired action toward your goals. Green aventurine supports growth in all areas of life, especially in the realms of career, finances, and personal development.

5. Crystals for Spiritual Growth

Spiritual growth involves connecting with your higher self, expanding your consciousness, and seeking alignment with the universe. Crystals that support spiritual awakening can help deepen your meditation practice, enhance your intuition, and open your mind to new possibilities.

- **Selenite**: A highly spiritual crystal, selenite promotes spiritual awareness and cleansing. It helps clear negative energy and opens up channels for higher guidance. Selenite is perfect for clearing blockages in your spiritual energy and creating a serene space for meditation or prayer.
- **Amethyst**: As mentioned earlier, amethyst is not only a tool for mental clarity but also a powerful spiritual stone. It enhances spiritual awareness and aids in connecting to higher planes of consciousness. Amethyst supports the crown chakra, making it ideal for those seeking to deepen their connection with their higher self or divine source.

6. Crystals for Creativity and Innovation

Creative growth is often a necessary aspect of personal development, as it allows you to think outside the box, solve problems in new ways, and express yourself authentically. Crystals that encourage creativity can help you tap into your inner inspiration and unlock new potential.

- **Carnelian**: Carnelian is a fiery stone known to enhance creativity, passion, and motivation. It stimulates the sacral chakra, the energy center associated with creativity and self-expression. Carnelian is perfect for overcoming creative blocks and reigniting the flow of inspiration.
- **Fluorite**: Fluorite is a highly protective and cleansing stone that promotes mental clarity and focus. It enhances cognitive abilities and stimulates the creative mind, making it a great choice for those working on creative projects or seeking innovative solutions to problems.

7. Crystals for Mental Clarity and Focus

Clear thinking and focus are essential for personal growth, especially when faced with life's challenges. Crystals that enhance mental clarity help you stay grounded, reduce mental clutter, and focus on what truly matters.

- **Lapis Lazuli**: This deep blue stone is known for its ability to stimulate the mind and improve decision-making. It helps enhance intellectual ability, aids in clear communication, and encourages self-expression. Lapis lazuli is also beneficial for expanding awareness and fostering mental clarity.
- **Clear Quartz**: In addition to supporting manifestation, clear quartz is also excellent for clearing mental fog and promoting focus. Its high vibrational frequency helps you align your thoughts with your intentions and clear any distractions that may stand in your way.

8. Crystals for Grounding

Personal growth requires balance between the physical and spiritual aspects of life. Grounding crystals help you stay centered and focused on the present moment, allowing you to take practical steps toward your goals without becoming overwhelmed by the process.

- **Hematite**: Known for its grounding properties, hematite helps to stabilize the energy body and promotes clarity of thought. It helps to anchor the spirit and provides protection from negative energies, allowing you to stay focused on your personal growth journey without distraction.
- **Black Tourmaline**: This crystal is renowned for its ability to protect against negative energies and ground the body. Black tourmaline helps you stay centered, both emotionally and mentally, and can be especially helpful when you are navigating stressful situations or making major life changes.

9. Conclusion

Crystals can be powerful tools for personal growth, supporting emotional, mental, and spiritual development. Whether you're seeking to heal from past traumas, boost your confidence, manifest your goals, or enhance your creativity, the right crystal can guide you along your journey of transformation. By selecting crystals that resonate with your intentions and using them regularly in meditation, self-reflection, or daily practice, you can tap into their energy and unlock your fullest potential.

Using Crystals to Aid in Spiritual Growth

Spiritual growth is a profound journey of deepening self-awareness, enhancing your connection with the universe, and cultivating inner peace. Crystals, with their unique vibrational frequencies, can act as powerful tools to facilitate this growth. By supporting clarity of mind, aligning the chakras, and fostering an intuitive connection to higher realms, crystals provide an energetic boost that complements spiritual practices like meditation, mindfulness, and prayer. Each crystal resonates with different energies, helping individuals access deeper levels of consciousness, spiritual insight, and overall well-being.

1. Crystals for Chakra Alignment

The chakra system, which consists of seven energy centers in the body, plays a vital role in spiritual development. Blockages or imbalances in these energy centers can hinder growth, while balanced chakras promote spiritual clarity and emotional well-being. Crystals that align with each chakra can help remove blockages, stimulate healing, and enhance the flow of energy.

- **Amethyst (Crown Chakra)**: Amethyst is a powerful stone for spiritual growth, particularly for the crown chakra, which is the gateway to higher consciousness. It promotes connection to the divine, enhances intuition, and brings clarity during meditation. Amethyst helps individuals tap into higher wisdom and opens them up to spiritual guidance, making it a popular choice for those seeking to deepen their spiritual practice.
- **Sodalite (Third Eye Chakra)**: Sodalite is known for its ability to enhance intuition and mental clarity, making it a valuable crystal for those working with the third eye chakra. It helps individuals trust their inner wisdom and promotes clear communication with the spiritual realm. Sodalite can enhance meditation, helping to quiet the mind and receive intuitive insights.
- **Rose Quartz (Heart Chakra)**: Rose quartz is a nurturing stone that activates the heart chakra, fostering love, compassion, and forgiveness. It opens the heart to unconditional love, not only for others but also for oneself. Rose quartz is often used in spiritual practices to promote emotional healing and create space for deeper connection with both oneself and the universe.

- **Carnelian (Sacral Chakra)**: The sacral chakra governs creativity, passion, and emotional expression. Carnelian is a vibrant stone that helps unlock creative potential and fosters a strong sense of self-worth. It encourages spiritual growth through self-expression, allowing you to embrace your true desires and passions.

2. Crystals for Enhancing Meditation

Meditation is a cornerstone of spiritual development, providing a space to connect with higher realms, clear the mind, and deepen self-awareness. Certain crystals can enhance the meditation experience by supporting mental clarity, tranquility, and spiritual connection.

- **Clear Quartz**: Clear quartz is known as the "master healer" because it amplifies energy, promotes clarity, and aligns all of the chakras. When used during meditation, clear quartz helps to quiet the mind, allowing individuals to connect more deeply with their spiritual self. It can also be used to amplify the effects of other healing crystals.
- **Labradorite**: Labradorite is a mystical stone that encourages spiritual awakening and expansion of consciousness. During meditation, it enhances the ability to access deeper states of awareness and helps to unlock hidden aspects of the self. Labradorite can be especially beneficial for those seeking to connect with their higher self or spirit guides.

3. Crystals for Developing Intuition

Intuition plays an essential role in spiritual growth, as it allows individuals to tap into their inner wisdom and guidance. Crystals that activate and enhance intuitive abilities can assist in making clearer decisions, understanding subtle energies, and receiving messages from the spirit world.

- **Fluorite**: Fluorite is a powerful crystal for mental clarity, focus, and intuition. It helps to clear the mind of distractions, allowing you to tune into subtle energetic frequencies. Fluorite is ideal for individuals seeking to enhance their psychic abilities and connect with higher realms.
- **Moonstone**: Moonstone is deeply connected to the feminine energy of the moon and is known for its ability to enhance intuition and psychic awareness. It promotes emotional balance and helps individuals tune into their inner voice. Moonstone is particularly helpful for those who wish to deepen their connection with their intuition and strengthen their connection to the divine.

4. Crystals for Manifestation and Spiritual Goals

Crystals are powerful tools for manifesting spiritual goals, such as developing higher consciousness, awakening to your divine purpose, and achieving inner peace. By programming crystals with your intentions, you can harness their energy to support the realization of your spiritual aspirations.

- **Citrine**: Citrine is a stone of abundance and manifestation. It is often used to amplify intentions and attract positive energy into one's life. For spiritual growth, citrine helps individuals manifest their highest potential, align their actions with their soul's purpose, and draw in opportunities that support their spiritual path.
- **Pyrite**: Pyrite is a stone of protection and abundance, and it is often used to manifest material and spiritual wealth. It can help individuals stay grounded and focused on their spiritual journey, ensuring that they align with their higher purpose while attracting the necessary resources to support their growth.

5. Crystals for Protection During Spiritual Practices

Spiritual growth involves navigating different levels of consciousness and encountering various energies, both positive and negative. Crystals that offer protection can help safeguard your energy and create a shield against negative influences during spiritual practices.

- **Black Tourmaline**: Black tourmaline is a powerful grounding and protective stone that is often used to shield against negative energies, psychic attacks, and environmental stress. When working with crystals for spiritual growth, black tourmaline can help to ensure that your energy remains protected and balanced, allowing you to move through your spiritual practices with ease.
- **Obsidian**: Obsidian is an intensely protective stone that helps to cleanse negative energy and create a shield around the individual. It can be especially helpful during deep meditation or spiritual work, as it provides a grounding influence and ensures that only positive energies are present.

6. Crystals for Connecting with Higher Realms

Spiritual growth often involves connecting with higher realms of consciousness, whether through meditation, prayer, or divine communication. Crystals can enhance your ability to access these realms and receive messages from the universe, spirit guides, or ancestors.

- **Lapis Lazuli**: Lapis lazuli is a stone of wisdom, truth, and spiritual awakening. It has been used for thousands of years as a tool to open the third eye and crown chakras, facilitating access to higher realms. Lapis lazuli promotes deep spiritual insight and enhances communication with spiritual guides, making it an excellent choice for those looking to deepen their connection to higher consciousness.
- **Celestite**: Known as the stone of angels, celestite is a gentle yet powerful crystal that facilitates communication with the divine and spirit guides. It promotes spiritual peace and harmony, helping you connect with angelic energies and higher

consciousness. Celestite can be used in meditation to open channels to the divine and receive guidance from higher beings.

7. Crystals for Grounding and Balance

Grounding is a crucial aspect of spiritual growth, as it helps individuals stay connected to their physical body and the present moment while navigating their spiritual journey. Grounding crystals can help keep you balanced, focused, and rooted in your spiritual practice.

- **Hematite**: Hematite is a powerful grounding stone that helps anchor spiritual energy into the body. It provides mental clarity and helps clear negativity, making it ideal for individuals who need to stay focused during spiritual practices. Hematite also provides a sense of stability and strength, helping to maintain balance during periods of spiritual expansion.
- **Smoky Quartz**: Smoky quartz is known for its grounding and protective properties. It helps individuals remain rooted while engaging in spiritual practices, ensuring they stay connected to the Earth's energy. Smoky quartz helps absorb negative energies and transforms them into positive vibrations, making it an excellent tool for both protection and grounding.

8. Conclusion

Crystals can be powerful allies in your spiritual growth journey, helping you deepen your self-awareness, enhance your intuition, align your chakras, and manifest your spiritual goals. By selecting the right crystals and incorporating them into your practices, you can foster a deeper connection with your higher self and the universe. Whether you're looking for protection, guidance, or balance, crystals offer a natural and supportive way to navigate your path of spiritual evolution.

Crystals have long been used to attract prosperity and abundance, drawing upon the energy of the Earth to enhance wealth, success, and overall abundance in life. Each crystal carries its own unique vibrational frequency, which can influence your energy field and help manifest positive outcomes. Whether for financial gain, opportunities or personal growth, certain crystals are believed to open pathways for attracting abundance into your life.

1. Citrine: The Stone of Manifestation

Citrine is often called the "merchant's stone" due to its association with wealth and prosperity. It is believed to carry the energy of the sun, bringing warmth, positivity, and abundance into one's life. Citrine works by helping you overcome obstacles and self-limiting beliefs, opening your mind to opportunities and possibilities. By stimulating the solar plexus chakra, citrine can increase confidence and motivation, encouraging action toward goals. It is particularly beneficial for those seeking financial success, career advancement, or business growth.

2. Pyrite: The Fool's Gold of Prosperity

Pyrite, often referred to as "fool's gold" due to its shiny, golden appearance, is one of the most well-known crystals for attracting abundance. This stone is believed to enhance wealth by stimulating the root chakra and creating a strong foundation for financial success. Pyrite is known for its energetic qualities that help draw prosperity into your life by boosting self-esteem and inspiring creativity. It also protects against negative energies and promotes a mindset of abundance, encouraging a healthy relationship with money.

3. Green Aventurine: The Stone of Luck and Opportunity

Green aventurine is considered a stone of luck and good fortune. It is often used by those seeking to manifest financial gains, career growth, or new opportunities. This crystal is known for its ability to attract prosperity through its stimulating effect on the heart chakra, which helps to foster an open and abundant mindset. Green aventurine is also believed to be helpful in overcoming obstacles, creating a positive flow of energy around you, and encouraging risk-taking in business or personal ventures.

4. Tiger's Eye: A Grounding Stone for Wealth

Tiger's eye is a powerful stone for manifesting abundance, particularly when it comes to achieving financial security. This crystal is known for its grounding qualities and its ability to balance the energies of the root and sacral chakras, making it an excellent stone for anyone looking to improve their material wealth. Tiger's eye helps increase courage and confidence, enabling you to make sound decisions that lead to success. Its ability to enhance focus and mental clarity also supports the manifestation of specific goals, helping you stay on track and avoid distractions.

5. Jade: The Ancient Symbol of Abundance

Jade has been treasured for centuries, particularly in Eastern cultures, as a symbol of abundance, prosperity, and good fortune. This stone is closely linked to the heart chakra and is thought to enhance relationships, which can play a significant role in attracting wealth. By promoting balance, harmony, and inner peace, jade helps clear the mind of stress and negativity, which allows you to manifest financial and material success. Many people use jade to attract favorable circumstances and maintain a positive outlook toward their financial goals.

6. Carnelian: Boosting Motivation and Confidence

Carnelian is a vibrant orange stone associated with creativity, motivation, and personal power. It activates the sacral chakra, which governs our passion, creativity, and ability to manifest desires. This makes it a potent crystal for stimulating abundance by boosting one's energy, passion, and determination. Carnelian can also enhance decision-making and help overcome procrastination, making it a useful crystal for anyone seeking to take action towards their goals. By raising your vibration, carnelian helps to attract opportunities for growth, success, and prosperity.

7. Malachite: The Transformation Stone

Malachite is a powerful stone for transformation, particularly when it comes to manifesting financial success and personal abundance. It is believed to absorb negative energies and transform them into positive, life-affirming forces. Malachite supports change and growth, helping you break free from limiting beliefs and patterns that might be holding you back from reaching your financial potential. By encouraging forward movement and resilience, malachite is an excellent stone for anyone looking to create lasting change in their financial or career pursuits.

8. Clear Quartz: Amplifying the Energy of Abundance

Clear quartz is known as the "master healer" due to its ability to amplify the energy of other crystals. When used in combination with prosperity stones like citrine or pyrite, clear quartz can help magnify their effects, attracting abundance more powerfully. It works by clearing blockages in the energy field, allowing the free flow of positive energy that can lead to financial gain and success. Clear quartz also helps to clarify goals and intentions, making it easier to stay focused on what you want to manifest.

9. Rose Quartz: Attracting Love and Abundance

Although rose quartz is often associated with love and relationships, it can also be used to attract abundance in a broader sense. By opening the heart chakra and fostering self-love, rose quartz promotes a sense of worthiness that encourages you to accept and receive abundance in all forms, not just financial. When your heart is open and you feel worthy of love and success, it becomes easier to manifest prosperity in various areas of life, including career, personal growth, and relationships.

10. Labradorite: A Crystal for New Beginnings

Labradorite is often called the "stone of magic" because of its mystical properties and its ability to open doors to new possibilities. It is particularly useful for those looking to attract new opportunities, whether for career advancement, financial growth, or personal success. Labradorite enhances intuition and mental clarity, allowing you to make decisions that align with your highest potential. It also offers protection, ensuring that your energy is shielded from negativity as you work toward your goals.

How to Use Crystals for Prosperity

To harness the energy of these prosperity crystals, it's important to engage with them regularly and set clear intentions. You can place these crystals in your home or workplace to attract positive energy, carry them in your pockets to stay grounded and focused on your goals, or meditate with them to align your energy with abundance. Setting a specific intention during your interaction with the crystals can also help amplify their effects. For example, holding a citrine while visualizing financial success or writing your goals on a piece of paper and placing it under a piece of pyrite can focus your energy on manifesting prosperity.

Conclusion

Crystals are powerful tools for attracting prosperity and abundance, helping you align your energy with the frequencies of wealth, success, and opportunity. By selecting the right stones and using them intentionally, you can create an energetic environment that fosters positive outcomes in your personal and professional life. Whether you're looking to manifest financial abundance, open yourself to new opportunities, or simply cultivate a mindset of abundance, crystals offer a natural and effective way to attract the prosperity you deserve.

Crystals for Goal-Setting and Manifestation

Crystals are powerful tools for enhancing the process of goal-setting and manifestation, acting as energetic catalysts that help align your intentions with the universe. Each crystal carries a unique frequency that can help you focus your energy, clear mental blockages, and empower you to achieve your desired outcomes. By incorporating these stones into your manifestation practices, you can amplify your intentions, attract the right opportunities, and stay aligned with your goals.

1. Citrine: The Manifestation Stone

Citrine is known as the stone of abundance and manifestation, often referred to as a "merchant's stone" due to its ability to attract wealth and prosperity. Its vibrant yellow energy stimulates the solar plexus chakra, which is associated with personal power, confidence, and the ability to take action. Citrine is particularly beneficial for setting and achieving financial goals, career advancement, and entrepreneurial endeavors. By placing citrine near your workspace or carrying it with you, you can boost your motivation, focus your energy, and create a positive, abundant mindset.

2. Clear Quartz: Amplifier of Intentions

Clear quartz is often called the "master healer" because it amplifies the energy of other crystals and can be used to enhance any manifestation work. Its ability to clear blockages and purify the mind makes it an excellent tool for clarifying your goals. Clear quartz helps bring your desires into sharp focus, ensuring that you are aligned with your intentions. It can be used in meditation or placed on an altar with written goals to amplify the manifestation process. When paired with other manifestation crystals, it helps to magnify their effects.

3. Tiger's Eye: The Stone of Confidence and Action

Tiger's eye is a stone of balance and courage, making it ideal for manifesting personal goals that require confidence, action, and determination. It activates the solar plexus chakra, which governs personal power and willpower, helping you overcome self-doubt and take decisive steps toward achieving your goals. Whether you're looking to improve your career, reach a personal milestone, or take on a new challenge, tiger's eye helps ground your energy and provides the confidence you need to move forward.

4. Rose Quartz: The Stone of Self-Love and Harmony

While rose quartz is primarily known for promoting love and compassion, it is also a powerful crystal for manifestation when it comes to personal growth, healing, and nurturing positive relationships. When manifesting goals related to emotional well-being, self-worth, or improving relationships, rose quartz can help you open your heart and build trust in yourself. By clearing emotional blockages and fostering a sense of love and acceptance, this stone helps create the right emotional environment to manifest your desires, ensuring they are in alignment with your highest good.

5. Amethyst: The Stone of Spiritual Clarity and Intuition

Amethyst is a highly spiritual stone that helps bring clarity and insight to your goal-setting and manifestation practices. By stimulating the third eye and crown chakras, amethyst enhances your intuition and connection to higher wisdom. This stone is particularly useful when setting spiritual or transformative goals, as it helps to clear confusion and align your goals with your higher purpose. Whether you're looking to deepen your spiritual practice, unlock hidden talents, or manifest personal transformation, amethyst provides the insight and guidance needed to stay on course.

6. Lapis Lazuli: The Stone of Wisdom and Truth

Lapis lazuli is a stone of wisdom, truth, and inner vision, making it ideal for manifesting goals related to personal growth, self-expression, and intellectual pursuits. It stimulates the throat chakra, enhancing communication, and the third eye chakra, boosting intuition and spiritual insight. Lapis lazuli is an excellent crystal for setting goals around creative expression, public speaking, or expanding your knowledge. It helps you stay authentic to your truth while manifesting success, ensuring that your goals are aligned with your deepest desires.

7. Green Aventurine: The Stone of Luck and Opportunity

Green aventurine is often called the "stone of opportunity" because it is believed to attract luck and new opportunities. This crystal is particularly useful when setting goals that involve financial success, career advancement, or expanding your network. Green aventurine works with the heart chakra to foster a positive and open mindset, which is essential for manifesting abundance. It is also a great stone for boosting your optimism, helping you stay positive and open to new possibilities as you work toward your goals.

8. Carnelian: The Stone of Motivation and Creativity

Carnelian is a fiery, energizing stone that stimulates the sacral chakra, promoting creativity, passion, and motivation. When manifesting goals related to personal projects, creative endeavors, or taking bold action, carnelian provides the energy and drive needed to stay focused and energized. It helps remove any procrastination or hesitation, pushing you to take decisive action and move toward your goals with determination. Carnelian is also a stone that fosters self-confidence, enabling you to trust your abilities and take risks that lead to success.

9. Sodalite: The Stone of Mental Clarity and Logic

Sodalite is a crystal that helps bring clarity and logical thinking to the goal-setting process. It is especially useful for setting goals that require mental discipline, focus, and analytical thinking. Sodalite stimulates the throat and third eye chakras, helping you communicate your intentions clearly and gain insight into the most effective path to manifesting your goals. If you have a complex or strategic goal that requires a clear, step-by-step plan, sodalite is an excellent tool to help you stay organized, rational, and focused.

10. Smoky Quartz: The Grounding Stone for Manifestation

Smoky quartz is a grounding crystal that helps clear negative energy and stabilize your energy field. It is particularly beneficial for manifestation because it helps anchor your intentions in the physical world, ensuring that your desires are brought into reality. Smoky quartz helps you release fears, doubts, and limiting beliefs that may block your manifestation process. It's also an excellent stone for staying focused and grounded as you work toward your goals, providing the emotional strength needed to overcome obstacles.

How to Use Crystals for Goal-Setting and Manifestation

To harness the full potential of crystals for goal-setting and manifestation, it's essential to engage with them consciously and intentionally. Here are a few ways you can use them:

- **Meditation**: Hold the crystal in your hand or place it on your body while meditating on your goals. Visualize your desired outcome and see it already coming to fruition.
- **Crystal Grids**: Create a crystal grid using your manifestation stones to amplify the energy of your intentions. Arrange the crystals in a pattern that resonates with your goals, and place them in a sacred space.
- **Affirmations**: Write down your goals or affirmations, then place the corresponding crystal on the paper. Let the crystal's energy support the manifestation process by amplifying your thoughts and desires.

- **Carrying Crystals**: Carry your manifestation stones with you throughout the day to stay connected to your goals. Simply keeping them in your pocket or wearing them as jewelry will help maintain your focus and intention.

Conclusion

Crystals provide a natural and powerful way to amplify your manifestation practices. By selecting the right stones and using them with intention, you can align your energy with your goals, remove blockages, and stay focused on your path. Whether you're looking to manifest material wealth, personal growth, creative success, or spiritual transformation, crystals offer a supportive and powerful tool to help you achieve your desires.

Crystal-divination Practices

Crystal divination is an ancient practice that involves using the energetic properties of crystals to gain insight, guidance, and clarity in various areas of life. This practice taps into the intuitive, vibrational energy of crystals to offer messages from the subconscicus, higher self, or even the universe. Much like other forms of divination, such as tarot or runes, crystal divination helps the practitioner connect to the unseen world, accessing deeper wisdom that can aid in decision-making, personal growth, and spiritual development.

Methods of Crystal Divination

There are several ways to use crystals for divination, each method having its unique approach and purpose. These practices rely on the crystal's ability to resonate with the energy of the individual or the situation, amplifying the connection between the conscious and unconscious mind.

1. Crystal Scrying

Crystal scrying, also known as crystallomancy, is a form of divination that uses a clear or reflective crystal to access visions, symbols, or messages from the spirit realm. To practice scrying, a diviner will typically gaze into a crystal, such as clear quartz or obsidian, allowing their mind to relax and focus. Often, the crystal may appear to cloud over, shift, or form patterns that lead to intuitive insights. The practitioner may then interpret these images as symbols or messages that offer guidance on a particular issue or question.

Clear quartz is especially popular for scrying because of its clarity and its ability to amplify the energy and intuition of the practitioner. Obsidian, with its dark, reflective surface, is often used to probe deep, hidden truths or to explore shadow aspects of the self.

2. Crystal Casting

Crystal casting involves laying out a variety of crystals in a specific pattern or arrangement, often called a "casting spread," and interpreting the positions of the stones to uncover meaning. Each crystal is believed to hold its own unique energy and symbolic associations, and their placement in the spread can provide insight into the situation at hand.

To begin, the practitioner may focus on a specific question or area of life and then toss or arrange the crystals in a random pattern. The interpretation of the spread relies on both the individual meanings of the stones and the way they interact with each other. For example, a cluster of citrine might indicate abundance, while a piece of amethyst might signal spiritual growth or mental clarity.

Some practitioners also use a grid system for crystal casting, where specific stones are placed in a set pattern, and the reader interprets the overall layout based on traditional meanings of the stones and their relationships within the grid.

3. Crystal Pendulum Divination

Using a pendulum for divination is another popular practice that involves crystals. In this method, a crystal is attached to a string or chain to create a pendulum, which the practitioner holds between their fingers. The pendulum is then allowed to swing freely, responding to the subtle energies in the environment and the practitioner's own energetic field.

Pendulum divination typically relies on yes/no answers or the identification of specific outcomes. For example, the pendulum may swing in a clockwise direction to indicate a positive response or in a counterclockwise direction to indicate a negative response. The practitioner may also ask the pendulum to point to particular symbols, directions, or numbers, which can then be interpreted to provide answers or guidance.

Common crystals used for pendulum divination include amethyst, clear quartz, and rose quartz, each offering different energetic qualities. Amethyst is believed to enhance intuitive insights, while clear quartz amplifies energy and rose quartz is used for heart-centered questions related to love or relationships.

4. Crystal Divination with Tarot or Oracle Cards

Many practitioners combine crystal healing with tarot or oracle cards to enhance the divinatory process. In this method, the reader may use crystals as an accompaniment to the cards, placing them on specific cards or areas of the spread to heighten the clarity and energy of the reading. Crystals are often selected based on their energetic alignment with the question or the cards drawn.

For example, if a tarot card related to career or success is drawn, the practitioner might place citrine or pyrite on the card to amplify its energy. For a card related to emotional healing or relationships, rose quartz or green aventurine might be used to reinforce positive outcomes.

Using crystals in conjunction with tarot or oracle cards adds an additional layer of depth to the reading, helping the practitioner tap into the specific energies associated with the stones. It also allows for more intuitive, energetic connections that can enrich the divination process.

Interpreting Crystals in Divination

Each crystal holds its own specific vibration, energy, and symbolism, which can be used to guide interpretations during a divination session. Here are a few examples of common crystals and their meanings in divination:

- **Clear Quartz**: Clarity, amplification, spiritual insight, and the clearing of blockages.
- **Amethyst**: Spiritual growth, intuition, and connection to higher realms, often used for guidance and wisdom.
- **Rose Quartz**: Love, self-care, emotional healing, and relationship matters.
- **Citrine**: Prosperity, abundance, confidence, and personal power.
- **Black Tourmaline**: Protection, grounding, and warding off negative energies.
- **Labradorite**: Transformation, magic, and spiritual guidance during times of change.
- **Sodalite**: Logic, communication, and truth-seeking, often used for decision-making.
- **Moonstone**: Intuition, dreams, emotional balance, and connecting with the divine feminine.

The Role of Intuition

In crystal divination, the role of intuition cannot be overstated. While each crystal carries specific attributes and meanings, the way they resonate with the individual and the specific context of the divination is crucial. Many practitioners rely on their intuitive abilities to sense the subtle energies that the crystals emit and interpret the messages accordingly.

Practitioners often report that as they become more attuned to the energy of the crystals, their readings become more accurate and insightful. Trusting one's intuition is essential in crystal divination, as the practice is not purely about following a prescribed set of meanings, but rather about connecting deeply with the energetic messages that are revealed.

Tips for Practicing Crystal Divination

- **Set Clear Intentions**: Before beginning any divination practice, it's essential to set a clear intention or question to focus your energy. This helps to align the crystals with your specific needs or goals.

- **Cleanse Your Crystals**: To ensure the energy of your crystals is clear and untainted by previous use, regularly cleanse your crystals. You can do this by using methods like smudging, placing them in the moonlight, or using salt.
- **Create a Sacred Space**: A calm and quiet environment allows for greater concentration and connection to the crystals' energy. Consider setting up an altar or designated space where you can work with your crystals.
- **Trust Your Intuition**: Don't rely solely on traditional meanings. Trust your inner guidance and let your intuition lead the way, especially as you work with the energies of the stones.

Conclusion

Crystal divination offers a unique and powerful way to access deeper wisdom and insight, allowing practitioners to use the inherent properties of stones to gain clarity and guidance. Whether through scrying, casting, pendulum work, or combining crystals with other divinatory tools, crystal divination can enhance personal growth, provide answers to important questions, and help navigate life's challenges. By tapping into the energy of crystals, you can develop a deeper connection with the universe and unlock hidden knowledge that can support your journey toward self-discovery and fulfillment.

Pendulum dowsing with crystals is an intuitive practice that combines the power of a pendulum and the energetic properties of crystals to access answers, guidance, and insights. This ancient divination method, known for its simplicity and effectiveness, has been used for centuries to locate hidden information, clear blockages, and provide clarity in decision-making. When combined with crystals, pendulum dowsing takes on an enhanced vibrational dimension, allowing practitioners to tune into both the pendulum's energy and the specific attributes of the chosen crystal to receive more accurate and powerful messages.

The Basics of Pendulum Dowsing

Pendulum dowsing involves suspending a weighted object—typically a crystal, metal, or other materials—at the end of a chain or string, allowing it to swing freely. The pendulum responds to subtle energy fields, moving in specific directions, such as back-and-forth, circular, or side-to-side motions. Practitioners use this movement to interpret answers to questions or gain clarity on various issues. The pendulum is often seen as a conduit, amplifying the user's intuitive energy and helping them tune into their subconscious mind, spirit guides, or universal energy.

The Role of Crystals in Pendulum Dowsing

The addition of crystals to pendulum dowsing can amplify the practice, as each crystal has its own unique energetic frequency. Crystals resonate with different energies and frequencies, which can influence the pendulum's movement in ways that offer more precise or focused answers. Crystals also help to fine-tune the energy of the dowser, allowing for a clearer connection to higher realms of consciousness.

Crystals such as amethyst, clear quartz, and rose quartz are commonly used in pendulum dowsing due to their specific energetic properties. For instance:

- **Clear Quartz**: Known as the "master healer," it amplifies energy and enhances clarity, making it ideal for dowsing practices.
- **Amethyst**: This crystal is used for spiritual growth, intuition, and accessing higher wisdom, making it an excellent choice for gaining deeper insights during pendulum work.
- **Rose Quartz**: Often used for matters of the heart, rose quartz supports emotional healing and can help with questions related to love and relationships.

By using different crystals for specific intentions, practitioners can tailor their pendulum dowsing to address various aspects of life, from health and career to relationships and personal growth.

How to Use a Crystal Pendulum

Using a crystal pendulum for dowsing requires a few simple steps to ensure that the process is effective and meaningful.

1. Choose Your Crystal

Select a crystal that resonates with the specific question or area of life you want to focus on. For example, if you are seeking answers related to love or relationships, rose quartz might be a good choice. If you're focusing on career or financial matters, citrine or pyrite could be more appropriate.

2. Set Your Intention

Before beginning, set a clear intention or question. The clearer your focus, the more likely it is that the pendulum will provide precise and helpful guidance. For example, you could ask, "Should I take this job offer?" or "Is this relationship serving my highest good?"

3. Hold the Pendulum Properly

Hold the chain or string of the pendulum between your thumb and index finger, keeping your hand steady but relaxed. Your arm should be supported, and you should be in a comfortable seated or standing position.

4. Ask Your Question

With your intention in mind, ask your question aloud or in your mind. Focus on the crystal, allowing its energy to align with your own. You may notice the pendulum begin to move of its own accord, responding to the energy of the question.

5. Interpret the Movement

Observe how the pendulum swings. Each direction can have a specific meaning, although these meanings can vary slightly depending on the practitioner's intuition and practice. Typically, these are the common interpretations:

- **Back and forth**: Yes or positive answer.
- **Side to side**: No or negative answer.
- **Clockwise rotation**: Affirmation or confirmation.
- **Counterclockwise rotation**: Rejection or negation.

It's important to note that pendulum movements can also be subtle. If you're unsure about the movement, take a moment to pause and re-center yourself before asking the question again.

6. Clarify and Confirm

If you receive unclear answers, ask the pendulum to clarify. For example, ask, "Can you show me a yes again?" or "Please show me a no." This helps to confirm the pendulum's responses and ensure accuracy.

Tips for Effective Pendulum Dowsing with Crystals

- **Clear Your Mind**: Before using a pendulum, clear your mind of distractions and negative energy. This helps to ensure that the answers you receive are clear and not influenced by external thoughts or emotions.
- **Cleanse Your Crystal**: Just as crystals can absorb negative energy over time, they should be regularly cleansed. You can cleanse your pendulum crystal by running it under water, using smudging herbs like sage, or placing it in moonlight.
- **Trust Your Intuition**: While pendulum dowsing can offer concrete answers, it is also an intuitive practice. Trust your inner feelings and interpretations, as they are often just as valuable as the pendulum's movements.
- **Stay Calm and Relaxed**: The clearer the connection between you and the pendulum, the more accurate the responses. Stay relaxed and allow the energy to flow naturally, without forcing the pendulum to move.
- **Use a Pendulum Board**: For beginners, a pendulum board with designated "yes," "no," and other markers can be helpful. This provides a visual guide and can make it easier to interpret the pendulum's movement.

Conclusion

Pendulum dowsing with crystals is a powerful and accessible method for receiving guidance, insight, and clarity on a variety of life's questions. Whether you're seeking answers to personal dilemmas, spiritual insights, or guidance on specific issues, the combination of a pendulum and crystal energy can enhance your intuitive abilities and help you connect more deeply with your own inner wisdom. As with any divination tool, practice and patience are key to honing your skills, but with time, pendulum dowsing can become a trusted and insightful part of your spiritual journey.

Scrying with crystals is an ancient practice that taps into the energy and vibrational properties of stones to access hidden insights and intuitive guidance. This method involves gazing into a crystal, allowing the mind to relax and become receptive to visions, symbols, or messages that arise from within or from higher sources of wisdom. Much like traditional scrying with water, mirrors, or fire, crystal scrying is a way to tune into deeper levels of consciousness, bypassing the logical mind to connect with the unconscious or the spiritual realms.

The Role of Crystals in Scrying

Crystals are believed to hold unique energetic frequencies that can amplify or direct the flow of energy. Each type of crystal has its own vibrational signature, making some more suited for scrying than others, depending on the desired outcome. Crystals such as clear quartz, amethyst, and obsidian are among the most commonly used in scrying practices due to their clarity, spiritual properties, and ability to act as a conduit for intuitive insights.

For example:

- **Clear Quartz**: Often used as a "master healer," this crystal amplifies energy, enhances clarity, and can help open the mind to spiritual messages. Its transparency makes it a popular choice for those looking for clear, unfiltered visions.
- **Amethyst**: A stone known for its calming and spiritual properties, amethyst helps to quiet the mind and connect to higher realms of consciousness. It is often chosen for scrying when seeking spiritual guidance or wisdom.
- **Obsidian**: Known for its reflective, dark surface, obsidian is a stone that is deeply connected to shadow work, protection, and uncovering hidden truths. It is often used for scrying when seeking deeper insight into personal challenges or unresolved emotions.

The reflective nature of these crystals helps focus attention and enhances the scryer's ability to access intuitive knowledge. As the scryer gazes into the crystal, they may begin to see images, shapes, colors, or symbols that provide messages or guidance related to their question or intention.

How to Scry with Crystals

While scrying is a practice that takes patience and skill, it is accessible to anyone who is open to intuition and willing to allow the process to unfold naturally. Here are the steps to begin crystal scrying:

1. Prepare Your Space

Find a quiet, comfortable space free from distractions. Lighting should be soft and gentle to help you relax and clear your mind. Many scryers prefer dim lighting or even candlelight to create a focused atmosphere. It's also beneficial to cleanse the space of negative energy before beginning, using methods such as sage, incense, or sound clearing.

2. Choose Your Crystal

Select a crystal that resonates with your intention. Clear quartz is excellent for clarity and general guidance, while amethyst is great for spiritual and emotional insights. Obsidian is ideal for uncovering hidden truths and protection. Hold the crystal in your hand or place it in front of you, ensuring that it is positioned comfortably for easy viewing.

3. Set Your Intention

Before you begin, set a clear and focused intention. This could be a question, a situation you are trying to understand, or a general desire for guidance. The clearer your intention, the more likely you are to receive meaningful and direct messages from the crystal. Be open to receiving any insights that come through, and allow your intuition to guide you.

4. Relax and Focus Your Mind

Close your eyes and take a few deep breaths, clearing any tension from your body and mind. Focus on your breath, allowing it to become slow and steady. Let go of any distractions, letting your thoughts fade into the background. When you feel calm and centered, gently open your eyes and focus on the crystal.

5. Gaze into the Crystal

Begin to softly gaze into the crystal. Avoid straining your eyes or looking too hard. Instead, let your vision soften, allowing the crystal to "pull" your focus. You may start to see clouds, patterns, or swirls within the crystal as you relax into the process. Some people report seeing colors, shapes, or symbols, while others may experience a sense of knowing or a sudden intuitive understanding.

As you gaze, try not to force any particular images or answers. Allow the crystal to guide you, and trust that whatever you see or feel is meaningful, even if it's not immediately clear. Some practitioners suggest asking a specific question in their mind as they look into the crystal, while others prefer to simply observe whatever images arise without focusing on a particular query.

6. Interpret the Images

As you gaze into the crystal, you may start to receive images, symbols, or words. These might appear as vivid pictures or as fleeting impressions in your mind's eye. Trust your intuition when interpreting these messages. If you're unsure, try to keep an open mind and note anything that stands out to you, even if it doesn't make sense at first. Over time, as you practice, you'll become more adept at understanding the messages that come through.

For example, you may see images of nature, such as water, mountains, or trees, which can symbolize emotions, challenges, or growth. Colors can also provide significant meaning—blue might indicate communication, green might suggest healing, and red could symbolize passion or energy.

7. Record Your Experience

After your session, it's helpful to take some time to journal about your experience. Write down any images, feelings, or insights that came up during the session, even if they seem unclear. This practice helps you process the information and gain a deeper understanding of the messages from your crystal scrying session. With time and experience, you may begin to notice patterns or recurring themes that help you refine your practice.

Tips for Effective Crystal Scrying

- **Practice Regularly**: Scrying is a skill that improves with practice. The more you work with your crystal, the more comfortable and attuned you will become to the energy and messages it provides.
- **Be Patient**: Scrying can sometimes take time to develop, especially for beginners. Don't get discouraged if you don't receive clear messages immediately. The process is about tuning into your intuition and trusting what comes through.
- **Trust Your Intuition**: The practice of scrying relies heavily on intuition. The images and messages you receive may not always make logical sense, but they often carry deeper meaning. Trust your gut feelings and the symbolic messages that arise during the process.

- **Use the Crystal's Properties**: Choose crystals that align with your specific intention. For example, if you are seeking insight into emotional healing, rose quartz or moonstone could be beneficial. For spiritual growth or connection with higher consciousness, amethyst and clear quartz are ideal choices.

Conclusion

Crystal scrying is a powerful tool for accessing intuitive insights, spiritual guidance, and deeper wisdom. By using the natural properties of crystals, practitioners can enhance their ability to see beyond the surface of a situation and uncover hidden truths. With practice and patience, crystal scrying can become a valuable part of your spiritual toolkit, providing clarity, direction, and a deeper connection to your inner self. Whether you're using it for self-discovery, spiritual growth, or guidance in decision-making, scrying with crystals can help illuminate the path forward.

Crystal healing tips:

- Cleanse your crystals regularly to keep their energy clear.
- Use saltwater to cleanse crystals, except for stones like selenite.
- Smudge your crystals with sage or palo santo to clear negative energy.
- Charge your crystals under the full moon for enhanced energy.
- Use a singing bowl or sound therapy to cleanse crystals.
- Place your crystals in sunlight to recharge their energy, but avoid prolonged exposure for sensitive stones.
- Meditate with your crystals to enhance focus and clarity.
- Program your crystals with specific intentions before using them.
- Use amethyst for spiritual protection and clarity.
- Place clear quartz near your workspace for enhanced concentration.
- Carry rose quartz for self-love and emotional healing.
- Use citrine to attract abundance and prosperity into your life.
- Keep black tourmaline in your home for protection from negative energy.
- Use lapis lazuli to enhance intuition and psychic abilities.
- Carry aventurine to promote luck and new opportunities.
- Place selenite in your home for cleansing and purifying the energy of a room.
- Use labradorite to help you connect with your higher self.
- Charge your crystals using sound waves, like with a Tibetan bell.
- Keep a piece of jade for good health and longevity.
- Use moonstone for balancing emotions and connecting with the divine feminine.
- Use carnelian for motivation, creativity, and boosting energy.
- Keep citrine by your front door to attract positive energy.
- Use tiger's eye for personal empowerment and grounding.
- Wear crystal jewelry to carry the stone's energy throughout the day.
- Use amethyst in your bedroom to promote restful sleep.
- Carry a piece of black onyx for strength and protection during difficult times.
- Use fluorite to clear mental clutter and improve focus.
- Use rose quartz in your workspace to foster loving energy.
- Carry turquoise to promote communication and creativity.
- Use garnet to boost vitality and passion.
- Place a piece of hematite in your home to ground energy.
- Keep a clear quartz cluster on your meditation altar to amplify intentions.
- Use green aventurine to heal the heart and attract love.
- Carry citrine to uplift your mood and energy levels.
- Use smoky quartz for grounding and removing negative energy.

- Place a piece of turquoise near your throat chakra to encourage clear communication.
- Use jasper to foster emotional balance and stability.
- Place a piece of malachite under your pillow to absorb its healing properties while you sleep.
- Use calcite to amplify the energy of other crystals.
- Place rose quartz in your bathroom for self-care and self-love rituals.
- Use moonstone for menstrual cycle balancing and fertility.
- Keep a piece of kyanite in your home for alignment and higher vibration energy.
- Use apophyllite to open up psychic channels and facilitate higher consciousness.
- Carry aquamarine for calm and peaceful energy.
- Use bloodstone for courage, strength, and vitality.
- Place black obsidian near you when doing shadow work to help uncover the subconscious.
- Use turquoise to cleanse and heal the throat chakra.
- Keep citrine near your workspace to promote productivity and creativity.
- Use pyrite to attract wealth and abundance.
- Use jade for emotional healing and cleansing.
- Use clear quartz in combination with other stones for stronger healing effects.
- Keep a piece of rose quartz under your pillow for dream work and emotional healing.
- Use amazonite to soothe anxiety and promote calm energy.
- Use ruby to ignite passion, motivation, and vitality.
- Carry amethyst for psychic protection during meditation.
- Use moonstone to balance feminine energy and intuition.
- Meditate with tiger's eye to boost self-confidence and inner strength.
- Place a piece of malachite in your home to absorb negative energy.
- Use aventurine for good luck and prosperity.
- Use selenite for protection and purification during meditation.
- Keep black tourmaline on your desk to absorb negative energy in the workplace.
- Use fluorite for mental clarity and problem-solving.
- Carry an obsidian stone when you need grounding and protection from negative influences.
- Use lapis lazuli for wisdom, clarity, and higher knowledge.
- Charge your crystals by placing them under the moon during the waxing phase.
- Keep a crystal grid to manifest intentions and enhance your healing practices.
- Carry rose quartz to nurture your heart and boost self-esteem.
- Meditate with a piece of amethyst to develop your spiritual gifts.
- Use citrine to enhance your manifesting abilities.
- Keep jade on you for prosperity and longevity.
- Use aquamarine for enhancing intuition and calming the mind.

- Use clear quartz to increase the flow of healing energy.
- Keep garnet in your home for vitality, passion, and strength.
- Use hematite to ground excess energy.
- Carry turquoise to protect your energy and foster good communication.
- Use labradorite to aid in spiritual growth and enhance psychic abilities.
- Place amethyst on your nightstand to promote peaceful sleep.
- Use moonstone for new beginnings and manifesting your desires.
- Use carnelian for inspiration and creativity.
- Use pyrite to protect yourself from negative energy and increase wealth.
- Use obsidian for deep healing and transformation work.
- Carry jade for healing energy, prosperity, and serenity.
- Keep a piece of selenite to purify the energy in your home.
- Wear a crystal bracelet to keep a stone's energy close to your body.
- Use lapis lazuli for deeper spiritual awareness and intellectual pursuits.
- Use rose quartz for healing the heart and fostering love.
- Use tourmaline for grounding energy and protection from negativity.
- Keep fluorite in your workspace to help with focus and decision-making.
- Use amethyst to calm anxiety and promote peaceful energy.
- Place black obsidian in a room to clear negative or stagnant energy.
- Meditate with a crystal to boost focus and inner peace.
- Carry citrine to keep your energy elevated and attract joy.
- Use sodalite for deepening your spiritual connection and intuition.
- Place aventurine on your desk to attract good luck and opportunities.
- Use carnelian to spark creativity and energize your goals.
- Keep rose quartz near your heart to invite love and harmony.
- Use garnet to increase motivation and personal strength.
- Use malachite to protect against environmental toxins and negative energies.
- Use apophyllite for heightened spiritual awareness and connection.
- Carry smoky quartz to absorb negative energy and promote emotional healing.
- Keep a selenite wand to clear energetic blockages in your aura.
- Use bloodstone for grounding and vitality.
- Keep citrine in your financial space to encourage wealth and abundance.
- Use amethyst for stress relief and emotional balance.
- Place jade in your wallet or purse to attract financial abundance.
- Use labradorite for spiritual protection and enhancing psychic gifts.
- Meditate with rose quartz for emotional healing and heart chakra work.
- Use tiger's eye for courage and mental clarity.
- Keep lapis lazuli near your throat to help with clear communication.
- Use fluorite to cleanse the energy of your environment.
- Place a crystal grid under your bed for peaceful and restful sleep.

- Keep a piece of jade by your front door for good luck and prosperity.
- Use amethyst to protect yourself from negative or toxic energy.
- Carry clear quartz to amplify the effects of other stones.
- Keep an obsidian stone near you when doing deep healing work.
- Use moonstone to aid in cycles of growth and new beginnings.
- Meditate with carnelian for energy and emotional release.
- Place turquoise under your pillow to enhance dream work and communication.
- Use selenite to purify and balance energy.
- Wear crystal jewelry to maintain constant contact with healing energy.
- Place a piece of fluorite in your work environment to improve focus and organization.
- Use aventurine to manifest personal growth and abundance.
- Keep rose quartz in your car to promote peaceful travel.
- Use clear quartz to help you focus on a goal or intention.
- Carry pyrite to protect your energy and attract wealth.
- Use black tourmaline to ground and protect yourself from negativity.
- Place amethyst near your computer or electronics to absorb electromagnetic stress.
- Use citrine to support decision-making and bring clarity to your life.
- Place carnelian on your sacral chakra to increase passion and creativity.
- Use lapis lazuli for enhanced communication and wisdom.
- Keep a piece of tiger's eye in your purse or wallet to attract prosperity.
- Use malachite for emotional healing and transformation.
- Place a rose quartz crystal near your bedside to nurture love and compassion.
- Keep a piece of labradorite near you to enhance your intuition.
- Use smoky quartz for grounding and emotional healing.
- Carry aquamarine to maintain calm and peace throughout your day.
- Place jade in your meditation space for emotional healing and prosperity.
- Use obsidian to connect with your shadow self and transform negative emotions.
- Use pyrite to shield yourself from energy vampires and negativity.
- Keep selenite in your home to purify the space and uplift energy.
- Use lapis lazuli to deepen meditation and spiritual practice.
- Use amethyst to reduce anxiety and stress.
- Place a piece of turquoise on your throat chakra for clearer communication.
- Use citrine to encourage positive thoughts and abundance.
- Keep carnelian nearby when seeking new ideas or creative inspiration.
- Use fluorite to cleanse your aura and remove energy blockages.
- Wear black tourmaline to protect yourself from electromagnetic fields.
- Use jade to maintain balance in your life and attract good fortune.
- Place selenite near your crystals to cleanse them and reset their energy.
- Use rose quartz to heal emotional wounds and promote self-love.

Have Questions / Comments?

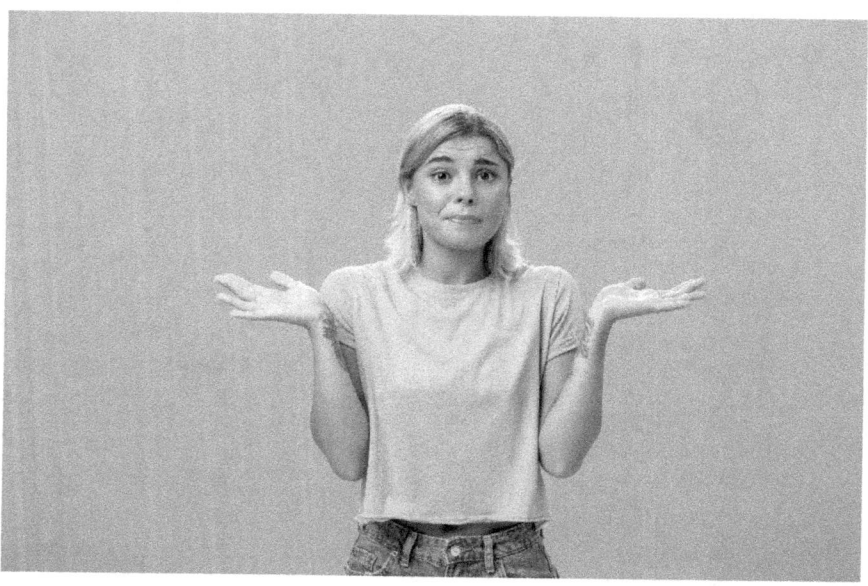

This book was designed to cover as much as possible but I know I have probably missed something, or some new amazing discovery that has just come out.

If you notice something missing or have a question that I failed to answer, please get in touch and let me know. If I can, I will email you an answer and also update the book so others can also benefit from it.

Thanks For Being Awesome :)

Submit Your Questions / Comments At:

https://questions.xspurts.com

Get Another Book Free

We love writing and have produced a huge number of books.

For being one of our amazing readers, we would love to offer you another book we have created, 100% free.

To claim this limited time special offer, simply go to the site below and enter your name and email address.

You will then receive one of my great books, direct to your email account, 100% free!

https://free.xsports.com

www.ingramcontent.com/pod-product-compliance
Lightning Source LLC
Chambersburg PA
CBHW052201220526
45471CB00004B/1766